THE CODE FOR WEIGHT LOSS

The Secrets Behind losing weight

By

Rafael P. Ray

Table of content

THE CODE FOR WEIGHT LOSS

Chapter 5

Chapter 6

Chapter 7

Conclusion

Introduction

Consequences of obesity

Individuals who have corpulence, contrasted with those with a sound weight, are at expanded risk for the vast majority of serious infections and medical issues. Likewise, heftiness and its related medical conditions monetarily affect the US medical care framework. Heftiness likewise influences military status.

Ailments

Stoutness in kids and grown-ups expands the gamble for the accompanying well-being conditions.

- Hypertension and elevated cholesterol are risk factors for coronary illness.
- Type 2 diabetes.
- Breathing issues, like asthma and rest apnea.
- Joint issues like osteoarthritis and outer muscle uneasiness.
- Gallstones and gallbladder illness.

Youth stoutness is additionally related with:

- Mental issues like tension and sorrow.
- Low confidence and lower self-detailed personal satisfaction.
- Social issues like tormenting and shame.

Heftiness as grown-ups.

Grown-ups with heftiness have higher dangers of stroke, many sorts of malignant growth, sudden passing, and psychological sicknesses like clinical despondency and anxiety.

Financial Effect

Yearly corpulence-related clinical consideration costs in the US, in 2019 bucks, were assessed to be almost $173 billion. Yearly cross-country efficiency expenses of heftiness-related non-appearance range between $3.38 billion ($79 per individual with stoutness) and $6.38 billion ($132 per individual with obesity).

Direct clinical expenses might incorporate preventive, symptomatic, and treatment administrations. Roundabout expenses connect with ailment and passing and incorporate lost efficiency. Efficiency measures incorporate representatives being missing from work for heftiness-related well-being reasons, diminished efficiency while at work, and unexpected passing and disability.

Military Availability

A little more than 1 of every 3 youthful grown-ups matured 17-24 is too weighty to even think about serving in the US military. Among the youthful grown-ups who meet weight necessities, just 3 of every 4 report active work levels that set them up for challenges in essential preparation. Therefore, just 2 out of 5 youthful grown-ups are both weight-qualified and satisfactorily dynamic for military help.

Additionally, 19% of well-trained help individuals had corpulence in 2020, up from 16% in 2015. These people are more averse to being restoratively prepared to convey. Somewhere in the range between 2008 and 2017, deployment-ready fighters had more than 3.6 million outer muscle wounds. One investigation discovered that deployment-ready fighters with weight were 33% bound to get this kind of injury.

Chapter 1

How Obesity turned into a plague

Weight reduction is a major business and since it's seldom fruitful in the long haul, it accompanies an underlying stockpile of rehash clients. What's more, specialists have been engaged with the business somehow for quite a while. About a long time back, the Greek doctor and thinker Galen analyzed "terrible humor" as the reason for corpulence, and endorsed back rub, showers, and "thinning food sources" like greens, garlic, and wild game for his overweight patients. All the more as of late, in the mid-twentieth hundred years, as scales turned out to be more precise and reasonable, specialists started regularly recording patients' levels and weight at each visit. Weight reduction drugs hit the standard during the 1920s when specialists began endorsing thyroid meds to sound individuals to make them slimmer. During the 1930s, the weight reduction synthetic 2,4-dinitrophenol (DNP) went along, trailed by amphetamines, diuretics, purgatives, and diet pills like fen-phen, all of which worked exclusively temporarily and caused incidental effects going from irritating to the deadly.

The public fixation on weight got a major lift in 1942 when a life coverage organization made a bunch of tables that turned into the most broadly referred to as standard for weight in North America. The Metropolitan Disaster protection Organization crunched age, weight, and mortality numbers from almost 5 million approaches in the US and Canada to make "alluring" level and weight graphs. Interestingly, individuals (and their PCPs) could contrast themselves with a normalized idea of what they "ought to" gauge.

Furthermore, look at what they did, utilizing progressively clinical-sounding terms like fat, overweight, and stout. The new phrasing supported the possibility that main specialists ought to and could treat weight issues. The word overweight, for instance, infers abundance; to be overweight recommends no doubt about its "right" weight. The word corpulent, from the Latin obesus, or "having eaten until a fat," helpfully conveys both a clinical environment and that intimately acquainted feeling of moral judgment.

By the 1950s, even as Hollywood glamorized well-proportioned entertainers like Marilyn Monroe and Elizabeth Taylor, medication was taking an alternate position.

In 1952, Norman Jolliffe, the overseer of New York's Department of Nourishment, cautioned specialists at the yearly gathering of the American General Wellbeing Affiliation that "another plague, albeit an old illness, has emerged to destroy us." He assessed that 25 to 30 percent of the American populace at the time was overweight or fat, a number he made up. "Nobody cherishes a chubby young lady except potentially a fat kid, and together they waddle through existence with a roly-poly family," composed Paul Craig, a doctor from Tulsa, Oklahoma, in 1955. Craig was enthusing more than a recent report that guaranteed "satisfying outcomes. On the issue of stoutness" by putting individuals on 800-calories-a-day consumes fewer calories and dosing them generously with amphetamines, phenobarbital, and methylcellulose. (Craig closed, in a remark that neglects to rouse trust in his strategies for logical request, "Not all individuals who eat ravenously develop fat, yet no hefty man or lady eats, as they guarantee, similar to a bird, except if they allude to a turkey vulture.")

In 1949, a little gathering of specialists made the Public Corpulence Society, the first of numerous expert affiliations intended to take heftiness treatment from the edges to the standard.

Through yearly gatherings like the primary Global Congress on Stoutness, held in Bethesda, Maryland, in 1973, specialists proliferated the possibility that managing weight was a task for exceptionally prepared specialists. "Clinical professionals deliberately showcased a defense that obesity was a clinical issue, and hence people ideally suited to mediate and gave viewpoints concerning it were people with M.D.s," says Abigail Saguy, a social scientist at the College of California, Los Angeles.

That's what those clinical specialists trusted "any degree of slimness was more grounded than being fat," composes Nita Mary McKinley, a teacher of brain science at the College of Washington, Tacoma. This demeanor propelled various new medicines for stoutness, including stereotactic medical procedures, otherwise called psychosurgery, which included consuming sores into the nerve centers of individuals with "net heftiness." Jaw wiring was one more obtrusive methodology that got some momentum during the 1970s and 1980s. It immediately become undesirable, perhaps because it quit working the moment individuals began eating once more. (Somewhere around one dental specialist in Brooklyn advances it.)

* * *

On a cool June evening in 2013, many specialists from around the nation spilled into the excellent dance hall of the Hyatt Rule Chicago. They were there, on day three of the American Clinical Affiliation's yearly gathering, to decide on a rundown of association strategies exhausting yet vital stuff, generally. Yet, one thing on the polling form that day would demonstrate quarrelsomely, and not simply inside the framed walls of the assembly hall. Goal 420 was short and forthright:

"That our American Clinical Affiliation see obesity as an illness level with different pathophysiological points requiring a scope of intercessions to propel treatment for obesity and counteraction."

The inquiry whether to group stoutness as an illness all by itself, or keep on thinking of it as a gamble factor for infections like sort two diabetes had been being talked about for quite a long time, both inside the association and outside it. Months sooner, the AMA asked its Board of trustees on Science and General Wellbeing to investigate the issue; the panel concocted a five-page assessment proposing that weight ought not to be formally named as infection, in light of multiple factors.

For a certain something, the board said, stoutness doesn't fit the meaning of a clinical sickness. It has no side effects, and it's not generally unsafe, for certain individuals in certain conditions, it's been known to be defensive as opposed to horrendous.

For another, a sickness, by definition, includes the body's typical working turned out badly. Yet, numerous specialists think weight the body effectively putting away calories as fat is an ordinary variation to a situation (times of starvation) that is turned out as expected for a lot of mankind's set of experiences. All things considered, the bodies that incline toward corpulence aren't ailing; they're more effective than normally lean bodies. Valid, we live in a when food is more plentiful for a great many people and life is more stationary than it used to be, and we don't have a similar need to store fat. In any case, that just method the climate has changed quicker than we can adjust.

At last, the advisory group stressed that medicalizing heftiness might hurt patients, making considerably more disgrace around weight and driving individuals into pointless and eventually futile "therapies."

The AMA enrollment disagreed with the board; they passed Goal 420 in a staggering voice vote.

I asked the association's leader, Ardis Hoven, an internist who represents considerable authority in irresistible sicknesses, to assist me with understanding the reason why the participants cast a ballot that way despite the board's proposal. She wouldn't converse with me straightforwardly, rather composing through a representative, "The AMA has long perceived corpulence as a significant general wellbeing concern, yet the new strategy embraced in June denotes whenever we've first perceived heftiness as an illness because of the pervasiveness and earnestness of stoutness."

There are, obviously, other potential clarifications for the AMA's choice. As James Slope, the overseer of the Anschutz Wellbeing and Health Center at the College of Colorado, told ABC, "Presently we begin getting a few normalizations for repayment and medicines."

All in all, follow the cash. Specialists need to be paid for conveying weight reduction medicines to patients. Coding office visits for Federal health care, for example, is a perplexing cycle that includes counting the number of substantial frameworks inspected and the number of sicknesses guided for if Federal medical insurance obliges the AMA and assigns heftiness as an illness, specialists who even notice weight to their patients could charge more for a similar visit than specialists who don't.

However, that is minor contrasted and such monetary irreconcilable situations shielded by some in the field. It's uncommon to find a corpulence scientist who hasn't taken cash from industry, whether it's drug organizations, clinical gadget makers, bariatric-medical procedure practices, or health improvement plans. The training isn't restricted to less popular lights, by the same token. In 1997, a board of nine clinical specialists tapped by the Public Establishments of Wellbeing cast a ballot to bring down the BMI cutoff for overweight from 27 (28 for men) to 25. Short-term, a large number of individuals became overweight, essentially as indicated by the NIH. The board contended that the change aligned BMI shorts with World Wellbeing Association Rules and that a "round" number like 25 would be simple for individuals to recall.

What they didn't say, since they didn't need to, is that bringing down BMI shorts, and placing more individuals into the overweight and large classifications, additionally made more individuals qualified for treatment.

Chapter 2

Acquiring Obesity

Obesity and Hereditary qualities

In the same way as other ailments, heftiness is the consequence of a transaction among ecological and hereditary elements. Studies have recognized variations in a few qualities that might add to weight gain and muscle-to-fat ratio dissemination; albeit, just in a couple of cases are qualities the essential driver of heftiness.

Polymorphisms in different qualities controlling hunger and digestion incline toward corpulence under specific dietary circumstances. The level of weight that can be ascribed to hereditary qualities changes generally, contingent upon the populace analyzed, from 6% to 85%, with the run-of-the-mill gauge at the half. Almost certainly, in every individual various quality add to the probability of creating stoutness in little part, with every quality expanding or diminishing the chances possibly, and together deciding how an individual answers the natural variables. Starting around 2006, over 41 locales on the human genome have been connected to the improvement of heftiness when an ideal climate is available. A portion of these obesogenic or leptogenic qualities might impact the hefty person's reaction to weight reduction or weight the board.

Qualities

Albeit hereditary lacks are presently viewed as uncommon, varieties in these qualities might incline toward normal stoutness. Numerous competitor qualities are exceptionally communicated in the focal sensory system.

A few extra loci have been recognized. Likewise, a few quantitative quality loci for BMI have been recognized.

A few examinations have centred on legacy designs without centering on explicit qualities. One investigation discovered that 80% of the posterity of two corpulent guardians was hefty, as opposed to under 10% of the posterity of two guardians who were of typical weight.

The frugal quality speculation proposes that because of dietary shortages during human advancement individuals are inclined to corpulence.

Their capacity to exploit intriguing times of overflow by putting away energy as fat would be favorable during seasons of shifting food accessibility, and people with more prominent fat stores would more probable endure starvation. This propensity to store fat, be that as it may, would be maladaptive in social orders with stable food supplies. This is the assumed explanation that Pima Local Americans, who advanced in a desert environment, fostered probably the most noteworthy paces of weight when presented with a Western way of life.

Various investigations of research centre rodents give solid proof that hereditary qualities assume a significant part in heftiness.

The gamble is not entirely set in stone by unambiguous genotypes as well as quality collaborations. Notwithstanding, there are still difficulties related to identifying quality cooperation for stoutness.

Qualities defensive against heftiness

There are likewise qualities that can be defensive against stoutness. For example, in GPR75 variations were distinguished as such alleles in ~640,000 sequenced exomes which might apply to for example remedial techniques against weight. Other up-and-comers against weight-related qualities incorporate ALK, TBC1D1, and SRA1.

Hereditary conditions

The expression "non-syndromic corpulence" is once in a while used to bar these circumstances. In individuals with beginning stage serious weight (characterized by a beginning before 10 years old and weight file more than three standard deviations better than average), 7% harbor a solitary locus transformation.

Proceeding with Schooling Movement

Weight is firmly connected to hereditary qualities and ecological elements. The most up-to-date examinations in the field of epigenetics further comprehension might interpret the impact of the climate on hereditary qualities. This article portrays the hereditary reasons for weight, including syndromic, monogenic, and polygenic causes, and refers to explicit instances of epigenetic adjustments related to heftiness. This action audits the assessment and treatment of hereditarily inclined weight and features the job of the interprofessional group in assessing and treating patients with this condition.

Goals:

- Portray the requirement for genome and broad affiliation studies to see better the way that weight can be acquired.
- Recognize the significant qualities related to syndromic and non-syndromic weight.
- Depict the critical times in human existence when epigenetic alterations can happen.
- Make sense of the significance of a definite history, actual assessment, and hereditary tests that can be utilized to analyze hereditarily and epigenetically acquired reasons for corpulence.

Presentation

The corpulence pestilence all over the planet influences grown-ups as well as youngsters. Around half of the time, corpulence in youth is conveyed into adulthood in a peculiarity known as "following." Per the most recent information from the World Wellbeing Association, the quantity of overweight and large youngsters under five years old is assessed to be nearly 39 million. In the US, 1 out of 3 grown-up Americans is large, and the Places for Infectious prevention has assessed that the predominance of weight among youngsters is 19.3% per information from the year 2017–2018. By 2030 a few disease transmission experts propose that 20% of the total populace will be large, i.e., having a weight record (BMI) over 30 kg/m² in grown-ups, or a BMI ≥95th percentile for age and sex in youngsters matured 2 to 18 years. Weight as an infection itself is multifactorial and happens because of complicated cooperations happening among hereditary qualities and the climate.

The Human Genome project was done between the years 1990 to 2003 to delineate the human genome. Expansive Affiliation Studies (GWAS) have been continuous starting around 2007 to assist partner explicit hereditary varieties with specific infections. Around 250 qualities are presently connected with corpulence. The FTO quality on chromosome 16 is the most significant and conveys the most elevated hazard of the stoutness aggregate.

The Hereditary Examination of Human Attributes Consortium is the association engaged with advancing exploration in GWAS. Nonetheless, hereditary changes alone can't make sense of the heritability of heftiness impeccably. The idea of epigenetics was acquainted with assistance to comprehend the heritability of corpulence better. Waddington previously presented the meaning of epigenetics was first presented during the 1940s by Waddington and in this manner expounded by Occasion in 1990. Be that as it may, the advanced meaning of epigenetics comes from Riggs et al. in 1996. Epigenetics is characterized as "the investigation of mitotically heritable changes in quality articulation that happen without changes in the DNA grouping." Epigenetic marks on the genome modify how every quality is perused to create an unmistakable aggregate. This gives a superior clarification of what the climate assumes a critical part in meaning how qualities are communicated.

Extensive Affiliation Studies (EWAS) started in 2013 to plan the epigenome and figure out the fluctuated articulations of qualities in various tissues. GWAS and EWAS have proclaimed another time in the investigation of hereditary qualities and weight.

Capability

Hereditary and epigenetic varieties add to stoutness by affecting the capability of metabolic pathways in the body and directing brain processes and craving focuses.

Consequently, these varieties impact insulin obstruction, dyslipidemia, aggravation, hypertension, and ectopic fat affidavit, particularly in the liver, which are the markers of heftiness. Hereditary changes can be acquired in an autosomal predominant or autosomal latent way and are impacted by hereditary components of erasure, hereditary engraving, and movement. Nonetheless, epigenetic alterations are more perplexing and happen at some random time and can be given from one age to another to cause corpulence. Geneticists have recognized a few pivotal periods when epigenetic changes happen, particularly during the development of the baby.

Factors affecting these epigenetic changes include:

1. Maternal nourishment both maternal over and undernutrition bring about epigenetic changes that can influence the hatchling and have intergenerational and transgenerational impacts. Maternal undernutrition and intrauterine development hindrance are known to be risk factors for extremely durable changes in fetal insulin digestion. Albeit this is an endurance variation system in fetal life, when these kids are conceived and presented to a supplement-rich climate, it inclines them toward fostering stoutness and type 2 diabetes. This idea is commonly known as the frugal aggregate speculation, which was advanced by Hales and Barker in 1992, and distributed in the Diary Diabetologia. The new phrasing for this idea is the "Formative Beginnings of Wellbeing and Infection speculation."

Human examinations that expounded this idea incorporates the Dutch Appetite Winter investigation of casualties of the Dutch starvation of 1944-1945, which took a gander at the progressions in the IGF2 quality, the Chinese starvation study, the Kiang West longitudinal populace concentrate on the Gambia, which took a gander at contrasts in populaces brought into the world in the wet and dry season with an extraordinary spotlight on the POMC quality. Maternal overnutrition, then again, including low protein and high-fiber consumes fewer calories, has been contemplated to cause fetal stoutness. The impact of maternal eating routine on fetal well-being is commonly known as the hypothesis of fetal programming. The rising pervasiveness of weight and type 2 diabetes in non-industrial nations like India and sub-Saharan Africa perplexed disease transmission experts for quite a while and is currently known to have its beginnings made sense by the hypothesis of fetal programming.

2. Maternal openness to poisons like organochlorines, polycyclic fragrant hydrocarbons, arsenic [which can cause gestational diabetes mellitus and subsequently fetal metabolic syndrome], and cigarette smoking can cause epigenetic adjustments. An illustration of this is changed in the GF11 quality found in moms who smoke >15 cigarettes daily. Specialists are presently naming these elements as "obesogens" or "endocrine-upsetting synthetic substances."

3. Maternal pressure has been related to diet-actuated corpulence in rodent models. The Quebec Ice Tempest Concentrate in people suggested the

relationship between type 2 diabetes and youngsters brought into the world to pregnant moms encountering misery after the tempest.

4. Maternal diabetes, more youthful maternal age, and low pre-pregnancy weight have been concentrated on in the relationship with fetal metabolic disturbances and later youth corpulence.

5. Nourishing aggravations in the post-pregnancy conditions and youth sustenance in twin examinations have been connected to adolescent stoutness and metabolic anomalies in early adulthood.

6. Changed stomach microbial vegetation with anti-microbial use in the primary year of life and, surprisingly, in adulthood is connected to heftiness and non-alcoholic greasy liver sickness (NAFLD). Microbial metabolites can cause epigenetic alterations, change quality articulation profiles, and cause genome reinventing.

7. Nourishment, overnutrition, prediabetes, and low protein consumption of fewer calories are connected to epigenetic changes related to fetal weight. There

is another interest in this field of "Fatherly Starting points of Well-being and Illness."

8. A high admission of sweet drinks, broiled food sources, highly soaked fats, rest aggravations, and a stationary way of life in adulthood has been connected to epigenetic changes.

In the research center, the well-evolved creatures used to study epigenetics incorporate sheep, pigs, mice, rodents, macaques, and drosophila. The tissues utilized in human epigenetic studies incorporate fringe blood-leukocytes and CD4+ Immune system microorganisms, rope blood, liver, pancreas, skeletal muscle, and subcutaneous fat tissue from the mid-region and butt cheek.

Issues of Concern

Hereditary Corpulence Can Be Delegated Monogenic and Polygenic Weight [included under nonsyndromic obesity] or Syndromic Stoutness

1. **Syndromic stoutness:** This can be additionally delegated corpulence brought about by chromosomal adjustments like Prader-Willi disorder, WAGR condition, SIM1 condition, and

pleiotropic disorders, including Bardet-Biedl condition, Delicate X condition, Cohen disorder, and so forth.

Prader-Willi condition (PWS) is brought about by the erasure of the Prader-Willi Basic District (PWCR) much of the time or by maternal uniparental disomy in 20 to 30% of cases.

The PWCR on the maternal chromosome is typically hereditarily engraved; consequently, the deficiency of the fatherly PWCR causes Prader-Willi condition. PWS is described by mental impediment, dysmorphic facies, hypotonia, short height, and hormonal lack notwithstanding weight. It is related to serious hyperphagia and food compulsivity in adolescence. The qualities in the PWCR that are lost incorporate NPAP 1, MAGEL2, SNURF-SNRPN, MKRN3, and NDN, which prompts lower articulation of proconvertase-1 in the nerve center, adding to heftiness.

Bardet-Biedl condition (BBS) is an autosomal latent illness seen more in families with a background marked by relationship. It is portrayed by issues in the BBSome, which is a unit of motility for cilia. Sixteen qualities have been embroiled in different types of BBS. Youngsters impacted by this problem present with learning disabilities, dyslexia, moderate bar cone dystrophy, hypogonadism, type 2 diabetes, labile way of behaving, renal anomalies, and polydactyly.

Different reasons for syndromic corpulence incorporate microdeletion condition, cancellation, Albright innate osteodystrophy related with GNAS transformation, Alstrom disorder ALMS1 change, Slashes disorder AFF4 change, Woodworker condition RAB23 change, Cohen disorder VPS13B/COH1 change, Rubinstein Tayabi condition CREBBP transformation, OBHD disorder NTRK2 transformation, Kleefstra disorder EHMT1 change, and so on.

2. **Monogenic stoutness:** Monogenic weight can be additionally arranged into autosomal prevailing or autosomal passively acquired types of hereditary heftiness. Monogenic corpulence by and large includes transformations in the leptin flagging pathway prompting concealment of anorexigenic and actuation of orexigenic pathways. To comprehend the many types of monogenic weight, it is pivotal to comprehend the unpredictable working of the leptin flagging pathway. Regularly, leptin follows up on the leptin receptor [LEPR], which expands the degrees of proopiomelanocortin

[POMC] and cocaine and amphetamine-controlled record [CART]. POMC, thusly, expands the degrees of proprotein convertase 1/3, which builds the development of alpha-melanocyte animating chemical [alpha-MSH]. Alpha-MSH then, at that point, follows up on the melanocortin 4 receptor [MC4R] in the nerve center to start the sensation of satiety. Additionally, leptin regularly smothers the neuropeptide Y (NPY)- agouti-related peptide (AgRP)- Y1R orexigenic pathway.

Autosomal passive legacy: Transformations in the leptin quality situated on chromosome 7, leptin receptor situated on chromosome 1, PCSK 1 situated on chromosome 5, and POMC situated on chromosome 2 are instances of changing qualities that have an autosomal latent legacy. Homozygous transformations in the leptin quality are by and large seen in consanguineous families and can be treated with metreleptin. Transformations in leptin receptors are frameshift, missense, or hogwash changes that can't be treated with metreleptin. POMC produces both alpha MSH and Adrenocorticotropic chemical (ACTH). Patients with POMC transformations foster focal adrenal inadequacy and skin hyperpigmentation. Transformations of POMC can be inactivating or garbage changes and patients can be treated with bremelanotide and hydrocortisone.

Autosomal prevailing legacy: Transformations in qualities SH2B1 situated on chromosome 16, MRAP2 situated on chromosome 6, and LPR2 situated on chromosome 2 are instances of changed qualities with an autosomal predominant legacy.

Transformations in qualities BDNF situated on chromosome 11, SIM1 situated on chromosome 6, and NTRK2 situated on chromosome 9 bring about unusual proteins associated with hypothalamic neuronal separation prompting the improvement of serious weight and mental hindrance. Transformations in MC4R have a codominant legacy and comprise the commonest reason for monogenic weight, with a predominance of 0.5% to 6% in various populations. Setmelanotide can't be utilized in that frame of mind of weakened or loss of capability of MC4R because its activity relies upon the typical downstream motioning of MC4R.

Other quality changes that can cause corpulence to incorporate NPY quality transformations, ghrelin receptor changes, MC3R quality transformations, and FTO transformations (the main quality changes adding to weight in grown-ups and kids).

3. **Polygenic corpulence:** A little over half of the acquired stoutness is polygenic. Polygenic corpulence is related to changes in CYP27A1, TFAP2B, PARK2, IFNGR1, as well as UCP2 and UCP3-which code for uncoupling proteins in skeletal and brown fat tissue, ADRB1-3 which code for the beta-adrenergic receptors influencing energy usage and lipolysis, and SLC6A14 which manages tryptophan availability for serotonin combination which influences craving control and energy balance.

Epigenetic Alterations Connected to Corpulence DNA methylation/demethylation-the most well-known component of epigenetic changes seen all through the genome. Methylation is represented by the activity of DNA methyltransferase 1 (DNMT1), and demethylation is completed by ten-eleven-movement (TET) compounds. Varieties in the methylation of CpGs in the genome comprise the "Differentially Methylated Areas" (DMRs).

Receptor change by acetylation and methylation. Histone adjustment manages five fundamental adipogenesis qualities, including Pref-1, c/EBP beta, C/EBP alpha, PPAR gamma, and aP2.

Histone variations: Histone macroH2A1.2 represses adipogenesis and increments leanness while advancing metabolic wellbeing.

ATP-subordinate chromatin redesigning buildings' association prompts further acetylation, phosphorylation, or methylation of qualities.

The expansion of miniature RNAs, long non-coding RNAs, piRNAs, or siRNAs prompts pre and post-transcriptional varieties in RNA.

Cross-sectional and longitudinal examinations have distinguished differential methylation destinations in CPT1A, ABCG1, and SREBF1 qualities in the blood, related to BMI variety. Differential methylation of LY86 in blood leukocytes is seen among corpulent and lean individuals. Variety in the abdomen to hip proportions differs with ADRB3 methylation in blood. Other critical epigenetic changes causing varieties in BMI have been seen in PGC1A, HIF3A, FTO, TCF7L2, FASN, CCRL2, and ELOVL2 qualities.

In pre-birth starvation, differential methylation in CDH23, SMAD7, INSR, CPT1A, KLF13, and RFTN1 qualities has been considered from grown-up entire blood tests. In intrauterine development hindrance, pancreatic islet disappointment and insulin opposition are connected to diminished acetylation of histones 3 and 4. Maternal high-fat weight control plans have been connected to fat tissue hyperplasia by diminished methylation of advertiser Scd1. Maternal corpulence has been related to hypermethylation of POMC in the fetal cerebrum and hypomethylation of dopamine reuptake carrier advancing fat and sugar desires in youngsters.

The stomach vegetation in grown-up life changes because of diet and can prompt epigenetic alterations like histone deacetylation and lower levels of methylation of FFAR3 and TLR. Accordingly, epigenetic varieties should be concentrated on unambiguous tissues because of the differential articulation of qualities in body tissues.

Clinical Importance

While diagnosing hereditary reasons for weight, great history taking, and actual test abilities are critical. A nitty gritty history incorporates individual history, family ancestry, medicine history, psychosocial history, diet and movement/practice history, and history of weight gain. Endocrine reasons for corpulence like hypothyroidism, development chemical inadequacy, hypothalamic weight, and Cushing's sickness should be precluded ahead of schedule with history, actual assessment, and lab work. Syndromic stoutness can now and again be particularly analyzed in light of the presence of actual elements, as in Prader-Willi's condition or Albright's genetic osteodystrophy.

After fundamental lab work is finished, including a total blood count, exhaustive metabolic board, development chemical, thyroid-invigorating chemical, and dexamethasone concealment test, doctors can check leptin, insulin, and proinsulin levels.

On the off chance that all the above blood work is negative hereditary testing can be completed.

These hereditary tests are costly and done in restricted focuses across the US. They incorporate linkage investigation to search for a familial collection of Mendelian characteristics, Sanger sequencing, chromosomal microarrays, cutting-edge sequencing with entire genome and entire exome sequencing, as well as intriguing variation affiliation tests.

The Food and Medication Organization (FDA) has endorsed two medications that target patients with hereditary reasons for heftiness metreleptin and bremelanotide. Different medications like semaglutide, liraglutide, phentermine-topiramate, and naltrexone-bupropion are endorsed for weight reduction in everybody and might be utilized to treat patients with hereditary stoutness.

Metreleptin is a leptin simple used to treat patients with innate summed-up lipodystrophy in leptin-lacking patients with transformations in the leptin quality.

In any case, metreleptin can't be utilized in patients with leptin receptor changes or transformations downstream in the leptin signally pathway.

The utilization of this medication is observed by the Gamble Assessment and Alleviation Systems (REMS) gathering of the FDA. The portion is by and large 0.06 mg/kg/portion once day to day for patients with weight <40 kg and 2.5 to 5 mg daily for weight >40 kg or grown-up patients.

Setmelanotide is an MC4R agonist utilized in fat patients with hereditary transformations in POMC, PCSK1, or LEPR qualities and Bardet Biedl disorder. The upside of this medication is that it acts straightforwardly on the MC4R receptor bypassing numerous objectives, which could be transformed in the leptin pathway. It is by and large managed as a 2 mg everyday subcutaneous portion.

Different medications concentrated in Prader-Willi disorder incorporate beloranib-a MetAP2 inhibitor and nasal oxytocin, however, these are not FDA supported.

Bariatric medical procedure with Roux en Y gastric detour, sleeve gastrectomy, and laparoscopic gastric banding has been displayed to help patients with hereditary reasons for stoutness.

The main exemption is in patients with a complete deficiency of MC4R capability where the bariatric medical procedure was not viewed as successful.

It is present all around concentrated on that particular medications can alter the epigenome of the body to help patients with heftiness. Instances of this are:

Bariatric medical procedures can cause changes in adipocyte-determined exosomal miniature RNA and cause epigenetic changes in differential methylated locales in HOXB1, PRKCZ, SLC38A10, and SECTM1 qualities.

Customary activity can cause boundless changes in DNA methylation in the RUNX1, NDUFC2, THADA, MEF2A, and PRKAA2 qualities. For patients who keep up with their weight reduction, the DNA methylation profiles look like lean people, as seen in RYR1, TUBA3C, and BDNF qualities.

Fasting can cause changes in DNA methylation of qualities LEP (leptin) and ADIPOQ (adiponectin).

The utilization of probiotics, prebiotics, and waste transfer can reestablish stomach verdure and cause positive epigenetic adjustments in patients with weight.

Different Issues

In broad affiliation studies done as such far, most subjects have European lineage.

Be that as it may, 47% or by far most of patients wrestling with the weight of stoutness in the US are of African-American and Hispanic/Latino plummet. The African Heritage Anthropometry Hereditary Qualities Consortium (AAAGC) and the Hispanic and Latino Consortium (HISLA) were made to concentrate on unambiguous alleles connected with corpulence in these populations. The Populace Design utilizing Genomics and The study of disease transmission (PAGE) concentrate on performed enormous scope genotyping including 54,000 members of African-American, Hispanic/Latino, East Asian, Local Hawaiian, and Local American plummet to concentrate on unambiguous hereditary variations related to stoutness.

The future of hereditary and epigenetics is promising, particularly in the space of heftiness and metabolic sickness. Epigenetics concentrates on the structure the premise of accurate medication with a particular focus on quality regulation. The reversible idea of epigenetic marks allows geneticists and clinicians an opportunity to propose changes in their way of life with dietary change and exercise and evasion of tobacco, liquor, and potential obesogens before patients and their posterity endure the side effects.

The utilization of histone deacetylation is currently being recommended past the limits of Hematology/Oncology for its utilization in way of life medication, and exploration in this field is continuous. Methylation Quantitative Attribute Locus (meQTL) studies are presently being utilized to facilitate epigenetic studies. New Nutri-pharmacogenomic studies are extending how we might interpret what sustenance means for hereditary qualities.

Improving Medical care Group Results

With the assistance of GWAS and EWAS, we currently figure out how hereditary qualities and epigenetics assume a significant part in heftiness. Diagnosing, making due, and supporting patients with hereditarily inclined stoutness requires a committed group of medical care experts experienced in their different fields with great cooperation. Starting from the beginnings of heftiness are straightforwardly connected with maternal well-being, a group of obstetricians, pediatricians, nutritionists, geneticists, and clinicians can assist with moderating gamble factors related to maternal and youth weight.

Pediatric endocrinologists assume a critical part in diagnosing youth stoutness. Interestingly, grown-up endocrinologists can help treat and control diabetes and other cardiometabolic boundaries that make epigenome changes passed on from age. The early way of life mediations, bariatric medical procedures, and prescriptions structure the premise of the therapy of hereditarily inclined corpulence.

Chapter 3

The Calorie-Decrease Mistake

Lessening Calorie admission may not assist you with getting in shape.

As it inclines toward numerous sicknesses and diminishes the future, the rising frequency of weight is among the best issues confronting humanity. By 2025, 18% of the world's male populace and 21% of ladies will be stout (NCD Chance Variable Cooperation, 2016): In the US 68% are now delegated overweight or hefty (Public Foundation of Diabetes and Stomach related Kidney Sicknesses, 2010). Endeavors to diminish heftiness have zeroed in on lessening calorie consumption, however, has an excessive amount of time been spent looking the incorrect way down the telescope? Is diminishing calorie admission prone to bomb as it disregards the instruments that the body uses to keep up with its current weight?

Mental mediations share practically speaking that they endeavor to lessen calorie admission, for instance attempting to control craving, increment satiety, or decrease segment size.

It has been guaranteed that "segment size is a modifiable determinant of energy consumption that ought to be tended to regarding the counteraction and treatment of weight" (Rolls, Morris, and Roe, 2002). It has been said that "food sources that objective inside dinner satiation and postmeal satiety give a conceivable way to deal with weight the board" (Halford and Harrold, 2012). On the other hand, exertion has been coordinated to figure out hunger, albeit an efficient survey neglected to track down a relationship between craving and energy consumption (G. M. Holt et al., 2017).

Attempting to decrease calorie admission is likewise the major rule that coordinates quite a bit of general well-being strategy. The U.S. government dietary rules recommend that we ought to "Keep away from larger than average parts." also the quantity of calories is imprinted on food marks and lower calorie choices are generally accessible in grocery stores. The U.K. strategy on good dieting proposes "putting calorie data on menus" and "assisting individuals with eating fewer calories (for instance by changing the piece size or the recipe of an item)." Notwithstanding, weight requests a more refined approach than counting calories: It should be treated as an interdisciplinary point.

Those offering mental guidance should be discerning of parts of both physiology and nourishment: Their proposals should be viable with real inclinations.

Scientists would in general look at physiological components that impact energy balance. For instance, the hypostatic speculation proposes that a middle in the nerve center screens metabolites in the blood and, utilizing critical components, endeavors to adjust energy admission and consumption. The methodology acquired a lift with the revelation of leptin, a chemical set free from fat tissue that decreases hunger. Conversely, analysts regularly expect the degree of muscle versus fat to reflect parts of the climate, food admission, or way of life. The current contention is that the interdisciplinary idea of stoutness requests the two methodologies: There are collaborations between physiology, the climate, and brain research. All the more explicitly it is contended that having a decrease in calorie consumption as the focal board of an antiobesity technique neglects to recognize the presence of physiological components that incline toward its disappointment.

Therapists keen on diminishing stoutness ought to think about changing their methodology. For what reason is a decrease in calorie consumption suggested when a lower energy admission prompts hormonal changes that invigorate hunger (Lean and Malkova, 2016), lessen metabolic rate (Dulloo and Jacquet, 1998), and animates the utilization of additional calorific food varieties (Benton, 2005)? Despite the fact that it might seem, by all accounts, to be the presence of mind to propose that eating less will diminish the gamble of gaining weight, this may not be the ideal methodology.

As the methodology taken by brain science is to decrease caloric admission, different inquiries are thought of. How does the body answer a little change in the caloric substance of dinners? How does corpulence create? What dietary methodology ought to be taken instead of essentially focusing on calorie consumption? At long last, with regard to the subsequent ends, how might clinicians concentrate on corpulence?

How Does the Body Answer a Little Change in the Calorie Content of Feasts?

Upholding a decrease in calorie consumption mirrors the understood supposition that physiological systems don't, to any extraordinary degree, balance energy admission and use. Notwithstanding, from one dinner to another and every day, food admission is described by extremely huge contrasts in the number of calories devoured. Prior to presuming that lessening the energy admission of dinners will be powerful, such changes should be put with regard to a great many social and mental elements. Moreover in the event that feasts differ enormously in size for a wide assortment of reasons, and transformations exist to streamline these varieties, changing the energy content of a dinner will have a restricted effect.

De Castro (1996) recorded food consumption for a week or longer. He saw that as numerous mental, social, social, and natural elements impacted the size of feasts, impacts that were strong albeit fleeting. The size of a feast was depicted generally as "unregulated," "flexible," and changing "precipitously inside a somewhat wide reach." Social help has an especially strong impact. He found that eating within the sight of one extra individual expanded calorie consumption by 44% while eating with six others raised it by 74% (de Castro, 1996). Moreover, acceptability, hunger, thirst, delight, and tension all impacted utilization.

Dietary restriction has been viewed as related to consuming 301 fewer calories daily in females (1.26 MJ; 16%) and 279 kcal a day in guys (1.17 MJ; 12%; de Castro and Elmore, 1988).

Confronted with these wide varieties in calorie admission, the significant inquiry is, how does the body answer? A shortsighted idea is that a calorie is a calorie and subsequently any raised admission of calories will bring about an expansion in body weight. Nonetheless, regardless of whether this was the situation, the effect of decreasing the energy admission of some food things will be restricted by the enormous impact of numerous social and mental factors. The effect will be even less if, over the long run, there are systems that smooth out the everyday varieties in calorie utilization.

Diminishing the size of dinners

Verifiable in the recommendation that lessening the energy given will assist with controlling weight is the view that the energy consumed in one dinner anily affects resulting utilization. Notwithstanding, over numerous years surveys have reached a similar determination:

Following a decrease in body weight, the lost energy is supplanted by modifications in physiology and changes in the idea of the food eaten (Drenowatz, 2015; Poppitt and Prentice, 1996).
Energy remuneration is more probable when you decrease as opposed to increment energy utilization. For instance, a review that endured 14 days, did a daze in a metabolic research facility, and tracked down that subjects "totally made up for the deficiency of calories." They expanded the number of food things devoured that contained ordinary degrees of calories. Conversely, they "neglected to make up for an expansion in caloric admission" (Foltin, Fischman, Emurian, and Rachlinski, 1988). Comparatively Drenowatz (2015) recognized that people are better prepared to shed pounds than keep away from weight gain, albeit the peculiarity is described by individual inconstancy.
Significantly, Poppitt and Prentice (1996) considered a period that prohibited any preload investigation of under 24-hr length. This time scale is significant as numerous mental examinations give

a dinner or a bite and afterward, after 120 or 150 min, measure food utilization.

This time scale isn't sufficient to permit full energy pay even though it has now and again been wrongly cited as proof that pay is of little significance. The time scale is basic as "energy balance in the lean is a drawn out peculiarity, molded by huge everyday changes in energy consumption" (Naismith and Rhodes, 1995).

The pertinent exploratory proof is presented by studies where obscure to the subjects, calories were eliminated from the eating regimen. It is fundamental, assuming you wish to show a reaction to changing the caloric substance of food, that reviews are done visually impaired: Purposely participating in a review produces general changes in conduct (Benton and Youthful, 2016). It demonstrated challenging to track down examinations that had clandestinely diminished energy utilization and observed ensuing calorie admission as most of the concentrates either had added calories or were not visually impaired.

Over a period as long as 24 days, following undercover energy decrease, all reviews revealed a level of energy pay that was differently 100 percent (Foltin et al., 1988; Lavin, French, and Read 1997; Louis-Sylvestre, Tornier, Verger, Chabert, and Delorme, 1989; Reid and Hammersley, 1998), 70% to 80% (Foltin, Fischman, Moran, Rolls, and Kelly, 1990; Porikos, Hesser, and van Itallie, 1982), or 40% to half (Naismith and Rhodes, 1995; Porikos, Stall, and van Itallie, 1977), even though it was just 16% in one case (Foltin et al., 1992). The most well-known reaction in these nine examinations was 100 percent energy remuneration. That is, lessening the calorie content of specific food varieties brought about no general decrease in energy utilization. However, on the other side there was a report of just 16% energy pay. Understanding these differential reactions might be the way to figure out how to profit from decreased calorie consumption.

Likewise, energy remuneration might be supported by changes in metabolic rate. For one day young ladies either abstained, consumed 1,200 kcal (5,040 KJ), or ate regularly; then for 4 days, they ate unreservedly picked dinners (Levitsky and DeRosimo, 2010). Body weight diminished altogether in the wake of fasting or confining the eating routine, although when permitted to eat typically the lost body weight was recaptured in 4 days or less.

There had, in any case, been no expansion in how much food is eaten, and it gave the idea that lessening food admission had diminished the metabolic rate and subsequently guaranteed the recuperation of body weight. This study recommended that the inability to keep a diminished body weight isn't guaranteed to mirror an expanded hunger or a raised food consumption; rather physiological components play significant parts.

With regards to endeavoring to diminish body weight, this is the absolute worst situation. For instance, when a bigger piece supplies more calories, on the off chance that it is important for a general and drawn-out expansion in energy consumption it will generally be put away as fat. The body doesn't attempt to diminish ensuing food admission to get back to the previous body weight but instead expects starvation by putting away energy. Interestingly, assuming calorie admission is diminished, the body remunerates by diminishing its metabolic rate or invigorating food consumption.

The transient guideline of energy utilization

Instead of expecting that diminishing calorie admission will impact body weight, a more modern origination is that there are administrative systems that impact future food consumption. At the point when food admission was estimated over days, de Castro (1996) tracked down proof of criticism systems. These components were said to act "quietly yet relentlessly," even though they were not evident for essentially a day, and typically a more drawn-out period was required.

An investigation of military students during essential preparation observed that on an everyday premise there was no connection between energy admission and use. Nonetheless, following 2 days in some, and a more extended period in others, changes were made (Edholm, Fletcher, Widdowson, and McCance, 1955). Again while cyclists partaking in the Visit de France were checked, the relationship between energy use and ensuing admission was nearer after 3 to 5, as opposed to 1 to 2 days (Saris, 1997). Both of these examinations analyzed genuinely dynamic people; be that as it may, a comparative finding has been accounted for in those showing more ordinary degrees of movement. At the point when food admission was recorded for a very long time, assuming there were deviations from the typical energy consumption, following 3 to 4 days there were pay in consumption that was not seen following 1 or 2 days (Whinny, Flatt, Volaufova, DeLany, and Champagne, 2008).

The discoveries are steady. Food utilization is affected by past energy admission, frequently after as much as 4 days. Hence transient examinations, of the sort that epitomizes a significant part of the mental work around here, will not be able to look at the instruments that control food consumption. The presence of components that smooth out everyday energy consumption proposes that the minor changes in caloric admission related to the adjustment of food things are probably not going to have a critical effect.

The More Expression Guideline of Energy Utilization

- **Counting calories**

What happens when, over a more drawn-out period, energy admission is decreased? Albeit an eating regimen might create a momentary increase, it is at a drawn-out cost.

Indeed, even one year in the wake of consuming fewer calories, the degrees of leptin, peptide YY, cholecystokinin, insulin, ghrelin, gastric inhibitory polypeptide, and pancreatic polypeptide have been found to vary from gauge values (Sumithran et al., 2011). That's what a survey reasoned "diet-actuated weight reduction brings about long haul changes in hunger stomach chemicals, hypothesized to lean toward expanded craving and weight recovery" (Lean and Malkova, 2016, p. 622). There are other physiological changes. At the point when food admission was limited, the subsequent loss of muscle versus fat was related to a decline in the creation of body heat and a decrease in metabolic rate (Dulloo and Jacquet, 1998), changes that will work with a re-visitation of the underlying weight. All the more, by and large, the apparent price of food expanded following weight reduction (Cameron, Goldfield, Cyr, and Doucet, 2008).

Given these reactions to counting calories, it isn't really to be expected that it has been recommended that in the drawn-out it doesn't work; any shed pounds tend not to be kept up with. Truth be told, an assessment of the drawn-out results of low-calorie slims down found that between 33% and 66% of health food nuts recaptured more weight than they lost at first (Mann et al., 2007). Weight cycling, or all the more informally yo slimming down, alludes to a pattern of weight reduction followed by recapturing the shed pounds, trailed by again counting calories, etc.

The Summermatter Cycle portrays how, at first during counting calories, the energy use of muscle lessens. In this way when more food opens up, the more frugal body leans toward saving fat (Summermatter and Handschin, 2012). Such a component shows that focusing on the decrease of food consumption, without understanding that the upkeep of weight reduction is significant, is probably not going to find success.

- **Weight vacillation**

Hence the body has as momentary objectives the streamlining of energy admission and keeping up with the current body weight. Nonetheless, in the drawn-out, different systems become possibly the most important factor that puts enormous fluctuations in weight down. Albeit over a time of months a lot of energy is consumed, over the long run there are in many cases somewhat little varieties in body weight.

The components are flawed, yet over significant stretches, the capacity of the body to adjust energy admission and consumption is faltering. It has been assessed that the normal 45-year-old male in

Western Europe consumes 1.24 million kcal (5,188 MJ) a year (Speakman and Westerterp, 2010). Correspondingly the Unified Countries Food and Horticulture Association determined that the normal American eats 3,790 calories (15.86 MJ) a day, a sum of 1.38 million (5,774 MJ) a year. Given food utilization information, the U.S. Branch of Farming found that for more than a year the typical American eats almost one ton of food.

Be that as it may, albeit an enormous energy admission may be supposed to be related to gaining a lot of weight, the figures don't make any sense. This degree of energy admission should be put about the U.S. Division of Agribusiness Dietary Rules. The association works out that an inactive grown-up male requires 2,200 calories (9.20 MJ) a day, which is 803,000 (3,360 MJ) a year. The equivalent figure is 2,800 (11.72 MJ) a day in genuinely dynamic people, amounting to a yearly admission of 1.02 million calories (4,268 MJ). Without the mediation of compensatory systems, this extraordinary abundance of energy consumption overuse would bring about a monstrous yearly increment of weight. An investigation of military students during essential preparation observed that on an everyday premise there was no connection between energy admission and use.

Nonetheless, following 2 days in some, and a more extended period in others, changes were made (Edholm, Fletcher, Widdowson, and McCance, 1955). Again while cyclists partaking in the Visit de France were checked, the relationship between energy use and ensuing admission was nearer after 3 to 5, as opposed to 1 to 2 days (Saris, 1997). Both of these examinations analyzed genuinely dynamic people; be that as it may, a comparative finding has been accounted for in those showing more ordinary degrees of movement. At the point when food admission was recorded for a very long time, assuming there were deviations from the typical energy consumption, following 3 to 4 days there were pay in consumption that was not seen following 1 or 2 days (Whinny, Flatt, Volaufova, DeLany, and Champagne, 2008).

The discoveries are steady. Food utilization is affected by past energy admission, frequently after as much as 4 days. Hence transient examinations, of the sort that epitomizes a significant part of the mental work around here, will not be able to look at the instruments that control food consumption. The presence of components that smooth out everyday energy consumption proposes that the minor changes in caloric admission related to the adjustment of food things are probably not going to have a critical effect.

Albeit these approximations can't be anticipated to deliver something besides unrefined appraisals, clearly the heaviness of the typical American isn't expanding by anything in the reach proposed by the contrast between the genuine and suggested degrees of energy admission. Without compensatory components each year, this distinction would bring about an expansion in weight moving toward 100 pounds.

The body weight of those in the Framingham Study expanded by a sum of 10% north of 20 years (Belanger, Cupples, and D'Agostino, 1988). In this way, somebody who was at first 150 pounds (68 kg) would 20 years after the fact be 165 pounds (75 kg); that is, the individual would have placed on 0.75 pounds (0.33 kg) a year. At the point when 15,624 Swedish ladies were checked north of 10 years, the yearly weight gain was 0.75 pounds (0.33 kg; Norberg et al., 2011). In a Scottish populace, north of 9 years the typical yearly weight increment, in those at first matured at 39 years, was 1.34 pounds (0.61 kg). Females mature at the first 59 years, expanding by 0.42 pounds (0.10 kg) a year, and guys by 0.20 pounds (0.13 kg; Ebrahimi-Mameghani, Scott, Der, Lean, and Consumes, 2007). Correspondingly north of 10 years a German report found a yearly weight gain of 0.55 pounds (0.25 kg) in guys and 0.53 pounds (0.24 kg) in females (Haftenberger et al., 2016).

With regards to the noticed yearly weight increment, it has been determined that north of a year 3,296 kcals (13.8 MJ) more energy would be consumed than had been used (Speakman et al., 2011). These figures mean a day-to-day overabundance of energy consumption over the use of just 9 kcal (38 kJ), a figure put in a setting by a teaspoon of sugar giving 16 kcal (67 kJ). Given the huge number of calories frequently consumed, factors other than calorie admission should be thought of.

There is, nonetheless, proof that the examination of weight change over significant stretches might deceive. Weight may not increment progressively, but instead stay stable for extensive stretches (Speakman et al., 2011), with weight gain happening now and again of extreme admission like Thanksgiving or Christmas (Yanovski et al., 2000). This perception of times of weight security again recommends a capacity to adjust energy admission and use. If for a significant part of the time the body can create energy balance, this would again contend against the assumption that diminishing the caloric substance of food will diminish body weight.

Normal changes in weight, notwithstanding, conceal individual contrasts. The Scottish example, for instance, revealed that the heaviness of 20% of the example changed minimally more than 9 years (Ebrahimi-Mameghani et al., 2007). Attempting to comprehend the reason why some figure out how to keep up with their current load while others put on weight might be productive.

A predictable picture has arisen. By and large, related to just little expansions in body weight. Obviously to comprehend the improvement of stoutness we want to look past the number of calories that pass our lips. The impression acquired is of finely tuned control components that screen and answer energy admission and use. Inspecting these control systems likely could be more useful than lessening the caloric substance of specific food things that are answerable for a little level of 1,000,000 calories.

How Is It Set in Stones?

A sufficiently based way to deal with managing body weight necessitates mirroring the components by which the body has not entirely settled and kept up. Two fundamental methodologies have been recommended: There is a "set" or a "settling" point. The set point hypothesis proposes that the degree of muscle versus fat is observed and contrasted and an objective worth (Kennedy, 1953). As required, admission or consumption is then adjusted to keep up with the ideal degree of muscle-to-fat ratio. One issue with this approach is that it doesn't make sense why the frequency of heftiness has expanded so extraordinarily. A subsequent issue is that it doesn't represent individuals with various ways of life having an alternate gamble of becoming fat.

Interestingly, the settling point hypothesis proposes that over the long haul body weight is connected with the example of food admission and active work into which individuals "settle" (Speakman et al., 2011; Wirtshafter and Davis, 1977). The organic systems that control energy balance are programmed by natural variables, to such an extent that the place where body weight is safeguarded may change over the long run. The settled point is shielded by metabolic and conduct variations. Rosenbaum and Leibel remarked, "The variety of frameworks directing energy stores and restricting the upkeep of a decreased body weight outlines that body energy stores overall and heftiness specifically are effectively shielded." The model recognizes that sustenance and physiology, as well as friendly, mental, and financial contemplations, all impact corpulence. Likewise, de Castro and Plunkett (2002) proposed that the guarded point reflects both the inward and outer milieu.

With the settling point approach, there is a need to recognize the underlying improvement of stoutness from resulting endeavors to decrease it. There can be no question that adjustments in the accessibility of food, and its expanded caloric substance, had a significant impact on the heftiness of pestilence. It follows that general well-being counsel has been to diminish food consumption, even though there has been restricted achievement. Sadly, albeit the elevated degree of calorie admission was a huge piece of the underlying issue, it doesn't follow that its decrease will be a significant piece of the arrangement. At the point when a decrease in calorie consumption has diminished body weight, there are strong physiological variations that favor recovering that weight (Scenic route, 2015). At the point when the underlying consideration related to endeavoring to shed pounds disperses, body weight increments and gets back to, or even surpasses, the beginning level (Mann et al., 2007).

Corpulence

The current contention that there are components that after some time safeguard the current body weight brings up an issue: If so, why would that be a stout pestilence? There are different contributory variables.

In the first place, stoutness frequently considers putting in a couple of pounds (0.5 to 1 kg) a year for quite a long time: that is, there is an excellent, but flawed, control of energy balance. Second, the idea of the whole eating routine is significant. To forestall energy remuneration, low-energy thick food sources ought to be eaten (see underneath). In any case, numerous Western weight control plans have a high energy thickness that quickly makes up for any decrease in energy consumption. Third, in numerous Western social orders, a significant indicator of corpulence is neediness (Drewnowski and Spector, 2004). Destitution is related to a low use of food, a low admission of products from the soil, and a high admission of fat. The least expensive food sources will generally have a high energy thickness.

One more piece of the response is that to control weight it should be feasible to both get thinner and keep up with that misfortune.

It is possible that it isn't the sum consumed at a feast that is significant but instead the absence of chance to forestall resulting compensatory changes. Having eaten a huge dinner, is there a potential chance to lessen calorie consumption in this manner? Frequently we don't eat because we are ravenous but since it is feast time; we don't pick what to eat yet rather eat what has been arranged by others; we devour not entirely settled by those serving the dinner, the food producer, or the food outlet. In that capacity, the chance to adjust energy utilization and consumption might be restricted.

Heftiness reflects many factors other than calorie consumption and any sound strategy ought to address more than the caloric substance of a feast.

If Not Calorie Decreases, What Approach Would it be a good idea for us to Take?

Although monitoring calorie admission is a methodology frequently taken by those in charge of their weight, the current inquiry is the degree to which lessening calorie admission can help all the more by and large to diminish corpulence. All the more explicitly, is clandestinely diminishing calorie levels, for instance by diminishing a piece size, going to be powerful in those not deliberately taken part in lessening admission?

The weight cognizant is effectively drawn in with attempting to not gain weight. As frequently these individuals are near energy balance, counting calories is possibly an effective methodology. There stay the 66% of the U.S. populace who are overweight while perhaps not currently hefty: In this situation, is lessening the calorie content of specific dinners supportive?

While the people who are weight conscious are working at the edge of energy balance and may try to consume less energy than they exhaust, the stout will generally have an admission in the abundance of use. As their admission is in many cases enormously in the abundance of consumption, over months a new and higher "settled point" is made. Why then should a little distinction in calorie utilization enormously impact body weight? The settled point is guarded, to such an extent that any abatement in energy admission will animate compensatory systems. In stout people, calorie admission will diminish weight provided that an energy deficiency can be accomplished.

Although both the large and the people who effectively control their weight are confronted with strong tensions to recover any lost calories, there are basic contrasts. Those keeping a low weight frequently utilize mental methodologies to forestall compensatory expansions in calorie utilization. The individuals who put on weight might know nothing about mental methodologies or may decide not to utilize them. Except if the hefty intentionally draws in with calorie control, requiring food makers and food outlets to decrease segment size would be inadequate. Assuming there is no cognizant control of calorie admission, the body will supplant the lost energy.

Furthermore, it is far-fetched that minor changes in diet will decrease the rate of corpulence, as controlling body weight will frequently require a total dietary makeover. It does, notwithstanding, appear to be probable that focusing on the idea of the food eaten, as opposed to just decreasing calories, offers benefits. A methodology that thinks about large-scale supplements, energy thickness, and glycemic burden might assist with forestalling energy remuneration.

Counts calories that help weight reduction

There are reports that craving, the control of body weight, and energy remuneration are impacted by the macronutrient synthesis of feasts (a measure of fat, carb, and protein).

At the point when in the transient the energy content of the eating regimen is diminished, assuming a portion of the accessible food varieties is energy thick, that is they give more calories per gram of food, then the lost energy will in general be supplanted. As a matter of fact, after lessening calorie consumption, just when the eating routine was consistent with a low-energy thickness was energy pay not noticed (Poppitt and Prentice, 1996). A meta-investigation of observational examinations observed that an eating regimen with a higher energy thickness was related to a higher weight record (Rouhani, Haghighatdoost, Surkan, and Azadbakht, 2016). As we will generally eat a comparable volume of food, a similar volume of low-thickness food varieties gives less calories. Hence a low-energy diet enjoys two benefits: It diminishes energy consumption yet in addition assists with keeping up with any weight reduction.

Low-energy thick food sources will generally have an elevated degree of water and a low-fat substance; products of the soil are genuine models.

A satiety file has been fostered that tracked down eating food varieties that contained more protein, fiber, and water brought about feeling more full after dinner, while the fat substance had the contrary effect (S. H. Holt, Mill operator, Petocz, and Farmakalidis, 1995). These discoveries were affirmed all the more as of late when 100 food varieties were evaluated for their apparent capacity to instigate satiety. Food varieties with a lower energy thickness, lower fat, and higher protein represented a large portion of the distinctions in the apparent capacity to prompt satiety (Buckland, Stubbs, and Finlayson, 2015).

A survey of the impacts of high protein eats fewer carbs inferred that there was "persuading proof that a higher protein consumption expands thermogenesis and satiety" and that "high protein dinners lead to a decreased resulting energy consumption" (Halton and Hu, 2004, p. 373). Eating protein animates energy consumption related to its ingestion, absorption, and digestion (thermogenesis):

This is assessed to be 23% of the energy consumed as protein, contrasted and 6% for starch and 1% for fat (Flatt, 1978).

In the wake of counting calories, in a randomized preliminary for quite a long time, either a high-protein or control diet was consumed. Satiety was higher and less weight was recaptured when high-protein dinners had been consumed (Lejeune, Kovacs, and Westerterp-Plantenga, 2005). Essentially, a Cochrane survey presumed that the overweight and large lost more weight when on a low-glycemic-load diet; that is, they consumed an eating regimen that delivered more modest expansions in the degree of blood glucose. It was noticed that there was a requirement for longer-term follow-up investigations to lay out a drawn-out benefit (Thomas, Elliott, and Baur, 2007).

In another review, overweight grown-ups lost 10% to 15% of their weight when they followed a low-sugar, low-fat, or low-glycemic-record diet (Ebbeling et al., 2012). The fall in resting energy use was, in any case, the biggest after the low-fat eating regimen: a significant perception as this would energize energy pay and the recovery of shed pounds.

In another review, subjects were checked for 7 days while secretly eating fewer carbs (Stubbs, Harbon, Murgatroyd, and Prentice, 1995). After a postponement of 3 to 4 days a more prominent admission of sugar or protein, yet not fat, was important for a negative input circle that decreased resulting energy consumption.

Subsequently, there is the possibility to foster an eating routine given the idea of the food things, as opposed to calorie content, that will assist with keeping a lower weight. Nonetheless, instead of focusing explicitly on the properties of individual food sources, it ought to be remembered that the routine example of eating inclines toward weight. Accordingly, an open door exists for brain research to energize the utilization of diets that are less inclined to be related to the acquiring or recapturing of weight. This will, nonetheless, include contemplations other than basically decreasing calorie admission.

Discussion

In outline, a momentary need of the body is to adjust the limits of energy consumption that happen from one feast to another.

Thus, minor changes in caloric admission are probably not going to have a drawn-out influence. A subsequent goal, following a deficiency of weight, is to guarantee a re-visitation of the previous body weight. These components have suggestions for those prescribing that we ought to attempt to lessen heftiness by diminishing calorie consumption: They recommend that the system, except if some portion of a more extensive intercession, will generally fizzle.

In the more drawn out term, the improvement of corpulence mirrors the evaluation by the body that, over a period, abundant energy had been consumed and consequently a new higher "settled body weight" is laid out. All things considered, it would be anticipated that the obvious cultural changes that brought about a positive energy equilibrium would result in a higher "settled" body weight; for instance, bigger piece sizes, eating all the more frequently outside the home, diminishing actual work, and the prepared accessibility of modest profoundly calorific food sources. If a set of experiences could be revised and these cultural changes switched, the opportunity for a more youthful individual to become large would decline.

Tragically, for the people who are as of now hefty, it doesn't follow that, without help from anyone else, diminishing calorie admission will prompt a lower body weight. The current body weight will be guarded.

Albeit the physiological systems that favor holding body weight are strong, this should not turn into a chamber of sadness. Maybe it ought to guide brain research to the assessment of parts of the climate and changes in conduct that can adjust their effect.

A conundrum

It might seem dumbfounding to propose that, while considering stoutness, consideration ought not to be coordinated basically to the admission of calories. We are, notwithstanding, battling numerous parts of current Western culture and substantial systems that have been created more than a huge number of years (Drenowatz, 2015; Scenic route, 2015; Poppitt and Prentice, 1996; Rosenbaum and Leibel, 2010).

In principle, the best technique is to forestall corpulence in any case by guaranteeing that no more energy is consumed than is used. Generally speaking, given the huge number of elements that impact the possibilities of accomplishing energy balance, such a goal will be accomplished solely after broad cultural changes. Subsequently, in expanding segments of Western social orders the body fosters a "settled point" that mirrors the degrees of energy info and consumption related to stoutness. How then, at that point, should the issue of heftiness be drawn closer?

By and large, a significant number of the endeavors to foster general well-being strategy can be summed up with the saying of the American columnist H. L. Mencken (1917): "For each complicated inquiry there is a response that is clear, straightforward, and wrong." It is indistinct why, as all serious specialists recognize that the starting points of corpulence are boundless and mind-boggling, general well-being drives would in general underscore a solitary or a couple of significant impacts. A genuine model was during the 1980s recognizing fat as the miscreant, with the outcome that general stores are currently overflowing with low-fat and "light" choices, yet stoutness progressed forward with a similar vertical direction. Along these lines, all the more as of late consideration has been paid by various gatherings to sugar, carbonated beverages, or part size. For what reason is it accepted that the starting points of corpulence are easy to the point that it will answer, even to a little degree, to secluded intercessions?

The public authority of the Unified Realm charged a gathering to frame the factors that lead to corpulence (Premonition, 2007). There came about a rundown of 110 elements that were gathered into eight classifications: food creation, food utilization, physiology, active work, energy balance, the actual work climate, social brain science, and individual brain science. Every one of these 110 elements was of impressive intricacy and portrayed by a labyrinth of criticism circles. Completely recognizing the intricate beginnings of stoutness underlines that it is generally impossible that the control of a couple of detached factors will have a huge effect. This isn't to imply that diminishing fat utilization or decreasing part size couldn't assume a part, yet just with regards to making changes to the whole eating regimen. Dietary methodologies can be anticipated to find lasting success just when part of a multi-layered, multidisciplinary enlivened mediation.

Clinicians need to invest more energy out of the research center as this area doesn't reflect a large portion of the variables that decide weight gain. The most vigorous of research facility peculiarities may not endure interfacing with the large number of elements that impact the propensity to gain weight. Most research facility reviews are speculation producing and before a methodology is prescribed it should be tried under certifiable circumstances.

Keeping a deficiency of weight

Although effectively controlling body weight is probably going to include a scope of drives, a significant number of which are irrelevant to food, the idea of the eating regimen assumes a significant part. The current investigation proposes that specific consideration ought to be given to endeavors to forestall the recovery of shed pounds.

It is not difficult to recommend that you ought to keep another lower weight however it is hard to accomplish. Getting thinner, contrasted with keeping up with weight reduction, is moderately direct. There are many various eating regimens, a large portion of which will find success, essentially for a brief period. In any case, of the people who lose 10% of their weight, just 20% will keep up with this misfortune for basically a year (Wing and Phelan, 2005). Accordingly, in the transient, it is feasible to keep up with weight reduction, albeit not very many will keep up with that misfortune for quite a long time.

The point ought to be to build this rate and to comprehend the elements that forestall the recovery of weight. What kind of conduct should be empowered?

Social changes

If lessening calorie admission isn't to be the focal driving rule, what is the other option? Over, a few methodologies were framed that could be utilized to foster a dietary style that will support the control of body weight. It would then should be shown tentatively that it worked. At last, the issue for brain science will be to guarantee its broad execution.

Key methodologies

The significant undertaking is to foster techniques that energize a consortium of social changes that understand the advantages of a suitable way of life. Dietary changes will be a section, however, a proper way of life and supportive character qualities likewise should be empowered (Wing, Tate, Gorin, Raynor, and Fava, 2006). A first undertaking will be to recognize pertinent parts of conduct.

Keeping up with weight reduction has been related to elevated degrees of active work, eating a low-calorie low-fat eating routine, having breakfast routinely, self-observing weight, keeping a steady eating design across non-weekend days and ends of the week (Wing and Phelan, 2005).

For any system to work it requires assessing the overall climate. At the point when investigations of well-being-related ways of behaving were likely to be meta-examination, different subjects arose (Kelly et al., 2016). Wellbeing related conduct was restricted by the strain of time because of family and work responsibilities, monetary expense, admittance to essential assets, low financial status, absence of information, and settled-in mentalities and conduct. Nonetheless, it was useful to zero in on happiness, have social help, coordinate new ways of behaving into one's way of life, and have an unmistakable message to follow. Any dietary mediation should be set in a social and social setting and the elements that work with or restrain the cycle should be recognized and reflected in a system.

Mental Commitment
Given the persistent physiological tensions to recapture shed pounds, the critical figure countering

these propensities is to intentionally draw in with the control of body weight.

As such brain research plays a specific part in recognizing and working with favorable mental styles and procedures. Keeping a lower weight has been related to expanded dietary restriction, seeing advantages as offsetting costs, having lower/stable degrees of sadness, and having a more sure self-perception. Correspondingly dichotomous reasoning, or at least, seeing things as limits, solace eating to direct state of mind, and disinhibited eating was pointless (Ohsiek and Williams, 2011).

As a capacity to screen the admission of food is a trait of individuals who effectively keep up with their weight over a significant stretch, it has been proposed that individuals may be prepared to self-manage, maybe utilizing controlled openness strategies (Johnson, Pratt, and Wardle, 2012). A survey of the best method for self-guideline saw that "higher independent inspiration, self-viability, and self-guideline abilities arose as the best indicators" of a gainful weight result.

These were accordingly proposed as potential targets while planning mediations (Teixeira et al., 2010).

One more synopsis of the region presumed that mediations that consolidated self-checking (following one's food-related conduct), gave input on execution, provoked a survey of conduct objectives, gave contingent prizes (compensating diet achievement), and made arrangements for social help were more fruitful (Prestwich et al., 2014). There was likewise proof that endeavors to oversee pressure worked on the progress of these methodologies.

In the executives' program an elevated degree of self-viability, the degree to which you accept you can achieve an errand, was related to the deficiency of more weight (Bas and Donmez, 2009). An assessment of endeavors to increment self-adequacy inferred that "activity arranging," "giving guidance," and "supporting exertion towards conduct" were related to more noteworthy self-viability, recommending approaches that could be taken (Williams and French, 2011).

Controlled eaters are people who watch their weight; they are ceaselessly worried about what they eat and attempt to restrict consumption. Ordinarily, their dietary limitations may not be sufficient to get thinner, however, they forestall weight gain.

A survey of imminent examinations found that controlled eating didn't foresee future weight gain, albeit the heaviness of the individuals who were counting calories was bound to expand (Lowe, Doshi, Katterman, and Feig, 2013).

One clarification is that health food nuts and limited eaters have a comparable propensity toward weight gain, albeit controlled eating all the more successfully kept it from working out. It is normal to propose that the progress of limited eating will be upgraded by the legal selection of food sources that consolidate a low degree of calories with the improvement of satiation, the inclination that the feast is finished, satiety, and how lengthy it is before you again wish to eat.

Chapter 4

Overtaking care of the Obesity

Refined how we might interpret the pathophysiology of corpulence. A portion of these experiences concerning energy homeostasis depends on the ID of new capabilities for peptides that were found many years prior. It is presently known that α-melanocyte-animating chemical, a peptide got from proopiomelanocortin and long perceived for its part in skin pigmentation through action at the melanocortin 1 receptor (MC1R), diminishes food admission and increments energy use through a connection in the nerve center with another melanocortin receptor, MC4R. In mice, designated erasure of the Mc4r quality outcomes in weight, hyperphagia, and hyperinsulinemia lessens energy consumption. Cancellation of Mc3r, the quality encoding a melanocortin receptor that is exceptionally communicated in the nerve center and limbic framework, likewise brings about expanded adiposity because of diminished energy consumption however doesn't cause hyperphagia.

Although powerlessness to normal stoutness is polygenic, transformations in MC4R are found in roughly 1 to 7 percent of people whose weight record (the load in kilograms partitioned by the square of the level in meters) is more than 40 and who become seriously fat before the age of 10 years. Opposition of anorexigenic (craving stifling) melanocortin signals is brought about by orexigenic (hunger invigorating) peptides, for example, agouti-related protein and neuropeptide Y, which are co-expressed in an alternate subgroup of neurons inside the nerve center. Agouti-related protein irritates the cooperation between α-melanocyte-invigorating chemical and MC4R, and neuropeptide Y diminishes the declaration of the quality encoding proopiomelanocortin (POMC). Different polymorphisms in the quality encoding agouti-related protein (AGRP) have been related either with security against heftiness or with anorexia nervosa. Neuropeptide Y likewise diminishes the union of thyrotropin-delivering chemicals and expands the amalgamation of melanin-concentrating chemical, another orexigenic peptide.

Circling convergences of leptin and insulin impact these focal components that control food admission and energy consumption.

The grouping of leptin in the blood is profoundly related to complete fat mass; stout people have high centralizations of leptin. The overabundant muscle to fat ratio that results from expanded leptin creation may be a revision for essential or optional disability of leptin-prompted signal transduction in the nerve center. The lessening in a muscle-to-fat ratio that happens with diet-prompted weight reduction makes leptin fixations diminish and sets off reactions that plan to moderate the muscle-to-fat ratio. At last, muscle-to-fat ratio mass mirrors the drawn-out balance between energy consumption and energy admission. The last option seems to play an overwhelming part in keeping up with this equilibrium.

How, then, do we choose when and the amount to eat? Long haul signals related to muscle versus fat stores are given by leptin and insulin. These flowing atoms likewise regulate momentary signs that decide dinner commencement and end. Signals that give transient data about appetite and satiety incorporate stomach chemicals, like cholecystokinin, ghrelin, and peptide YY3-36 (PYY), and signals from vagal afferent neurons inside the gastrointestinal lot that answer mechanical distortion, macronutrients, pH, constitution, and chemicals.

Brain and humoral signs are then coordinated in unambiguous districts of the nerve center and cerebrum stem.

In this issue of the Diary Batterham et al. report an investigation of PYY, a peptide that is discharged postprandially, concerning the calories ingested, by endocrine L cells coating the distal little gut and colon. The examiners tracked down that a solitary imbuement of PYY, as contrasted and a mixture of saline, decreased hunger and food utilization by roughly 30% at an all-you-need-to-have buffet lunch given two hours after the implantation. In the hefty subjects, the endogenous postprandial PYY reaction was lessened as contrasted with that in the lean subjects, even though the stout subjects consumed a more noteworthy number of calories. The PYY mixture decreased hunger in both the hefty and lean gatherings and meaningfully affected subjects' reports of the acceptability of the feasts or their sensations of sickness.

The underlying arrival of PYY happens soon after food consumption, apparently through brain components, before ingested supplements show up in the distal part of the small digestive tract and the colon.

The resulting arrival of PYY is animated by supplements, especially sugars and lipids, inside the lumen of the distal piece of the small digestive system and the colon. PYY diminishes food consumption through restraint of stomach motility (going about as an "ileal brake" to cause a feeling of satiety) and via vagal afferent neurons that rise from the gastrointestinal parcel to the hindbrain and collaborations with humoral receptors in the nerve center. In examinations in creatures, PYY hindered the hypothalamic neuropeptide Y-communicating neurons and agouti-related protein-communicating neurons through inhibitory neuropeptide Y2 receptors, subsequently disinhibiting contiguous proopiomelanocortin-communicating neurons and diminishing food admission.

The concentrate by Batterham et al. additionally shows that implantation of PYY diminishes fasting groupings of the orexigenic peptide ghrelin. Ghrelin is a 28-amino-corrosive, acylated peptide discharged by oxyntic cells in the stomach fundus. Ghrelin follows up on the development of chemical secretagogue receptors to expand the arrival of development chemicals from the pituitary.

As of late, the putative jobs of ghrelin in energy homeostasis and, specifically, premeal appetite and dinner commencement have been distinguished. Flowing ghrelin focuses on increment preprandial and decline postprandially. Ghrelin increases food consumption through the feeling of ghrelin receptors on hypothalamic neuropeptide Y-communicating neurons and agouti-related protein-communicating neurons. Although the PYY mixture lessens the groupings of ghrelin in lean and stout subjects who are fasting and decreases the preprandial ascent in ghrelin in lean subjects, the degree to which concealment of ghrelin discharge adds to a PYY-interceded decrease in food admission is hazy.

Assuming ghrelin signals hunger and PYY signals satiety, might these chemicals at any point be controlled restoratively? Quality knockout examinations in mice uncover that one can only with significant effort fool the homeostatic components that keep up with muscle versus fat: exploratory knockouts of the ghrelin quality, AgRP, and the neuropeptide Y quality (Npy) and a twofold knockout of AgRP and Npy are not related with any undeniable impacts on energy digestion of food consumption. Conversely, inactivating transformations of POMC, the qualities that encode leptin and the leptin receptor, and MC4R produce significant fat aggregates in mice as well as in people. Orexigenic pathways are so basic to endurance that the shortfall of one peptide is made up for by the activities of others. Investigations of stomach chemicals after weight reduction prompted by consuming fewer calories or medical procedures have given a few insights into likely pharmacologic treatments. Weight reduction by caloric limitation is related to an expansion in hunger and flowing centralizations of ghrelin. After gastric detour a medical procedure, hunger lessens, flowing groupings of ghrelin decline, and circling centralizations of PYY increment. Hormonal changes after sidestepping a medical procedure may in this manner have an impact on the concealment of yearning and the drawn-out upkeep of diminished body weight.

Albeit single intraperitoneal infusions of PYY decline food consumption for as long as seven days in rodents, the consequences of solitary implantation in people can't be extrapolated to anticipate long-haul results. The utilization of PYY might keep counterregulatory instruments from superseding the feeling of anorexigenic pathways.

Nonetheless, the improvement of antibodies or tachyphylaxis through receptor down-guideline might restrict the viability of drawn-out PYY organization. No one particle or subordinate may give an enchanted projectile to initiate and keep up with weight reduction. Fruitful pharmacologic treatment for weight might be conceivable exclusively by at the same time focusing on the interlocking, repetitive frameworks that drive food admission and act to oppose the deficiency of muscle-to-fat ratio.

Chapter 5

Fats that make you fat, fats that make you lean

Solid Fats: Your Complete Rundown

Fat was the miscreant for a long time. The standard exhortation to general society was to diminish fat admission to shed pounds and further develop well-being. That exhortation ended up being generally off-base.

It just so happens, not all fat is something very similar, a low-fat eating routine isn't the main way, or even the most effective way, to get more fit and further develop well-being. A superior way to deal with hitting your objectives might be to pick specific sorts of fat known to have medical advantages. This is some data on the best way to make fat your companion for diabetes anticipation and weight reduction.

Sorts of Fat

Dietary fat is a supplement in numerous food sources. It gives around 9 calories for each gram, which is over two times the 4 calories for every gram that protein and starches contain.

Consequently, fats and high-fat food varieties are high in calories. It is not difficult to get a lot of calories rapidly from fat and high-fat food varieties.

Be that as it may, there are many kinds of dietary fat, and they contrastingly affect your well-being. A few kinds of fat advance heart well-being and are connected to weight reduction and lower diabetes risk. Different fats make the contrary difference.

Bad Fats

Generally immersed and trans fats are viewed as unfortunate fats. Creature fats, like in greasy red meat, spread, and poultry skin, are wealthy in immersed fat. They might be terrible for your heart, weight, insulin awareness, and diabetes risk. By and large, intend to keep your admission of soaked fats to under 7 to 10% of complete calories, or 16 to 22 grams each day on a 2,000-calorie diet.

Tropical oils, for example, palm oil and coconut oil, are likewise high in immersed fat. Certain individuals are defenders of coconut oil as sound fat, albeit most proof shows that coconut oil is undesirable. The kinds of soaked fat in dairy items and chocolate don't seem to hurtfully affect your well-being.

Trans fats give off an impression of being the most terrible sort of fat. Indeed, even two or three grams each day can be unsafe. They can raise "awful" LDL cholesterol, lower "great" HDL cholesterol, raise coronary illness risk, hinder insulin activity, and increase your gamble for diabetes. You are best off keeping away from trans fats however much as could reasonably be expected, with an objective of zero grams every day.

Some trans fats are normally tracked down in red meat, however, these don't seem, by all accounts, to be unsafe. Interestingly, counterfeit trans fats that are created while searing or during food handling are the hurtful ones. You can keep away from counterfeit trans fats by skirting broiled food varieties and keeping away from handled food sources with fixings like to some extent hydrogenated oil.

Utilize fat for your potential benefit
Supplant bad fats with great ones.
Pick cooking strategies other than broiling.
Keep segment estimates little, like an ounce of nuts or a teaspoon of oil.
Decrease carbs a little by diminishing refined starches and sugars (white bread, sugar food sources) and expanding sound fats. For instance, rather than a two-piece sandwich shut face, have one piece open-confronted with a cut of avocado.
Pick fish rather than red meat here and there.
Utilize fat for your potential benefit
Supplant terrible fats with great ones.
Pick cooking strategies other than broiling.
Keep segment estimates little, like an ounce of nuts or a teaspoon of oil.
Lessen carbs a little by diminishing refined starches and sugars (white bread, sugar food sources) and expanding sound fats. For instance, rather than a two-piece sandwich shut face, have one piece open-confronted with a cut of avocado.

Pick fish rather than red meat at times.

Great Fats - Omega-3, 6, and 9's
Why Fish Is a Sound Protein, And How To Get A greater amount of It
The "upside" fats are connected to medical advantages including lower body weight and lower risk for coronary illness and diabetes., They will quite often be unsaturated fats, including monounsaturated fats and polyunsaturated fats.

Monounsaturated fats, at times called MUFA, are omega-9 fats.

They are known for their job in heart well-being and their presence in Mediterranean-style abstains from food. These popular fats might bring down pulse, fatty oils, aggregate and "terrible" LDL cholesterol, and diabetes risk. Sources incorporate avocados, olive oil, nuts, and peanuts.

Polyunsaturated fats incorporate omega-6 and omega-3 fats. The omega-3 fats are heart-sound, with impacts, for example, bringing down pulse, forestalling blood clumps, battling aggravation, and expanding "great" HDL cholesterol. Omega-3's are great for the mind and your temperament, and they can bring down diabetes risk. They might try and assist you with controlling your weight.

Fish is a wellspring of long-chain omega-3 fats known as EPA and DHA. The best sources are greasy fish, like trout, sardines, anchovies, herring, fish, mackerel, and salmon. On the off chance that you stay away from fish, you can get some omega-3s, in a structure known as ALA, from pecans and flaxseed. Be that as it may, your body can change over a restricted measure of ALA into DHA. A decent objective is to have fish two times per week to get sufficient EPA and DHA.

Omega-6 fats can make a few unfortunate favorable to incendiary impacts, and a few sound-calming impacts. They are not difficult to get into the American eating regimen, with vegetable oils and nuts being rich sources.
The way to omega-6 fats isn't to have them excessively. You are best off adding omega-6 fats into your eating regimen not as an option, yet rather as a substitute for fewer sound decisions, like soaked fats and refined starches. For instance, you can utilize sunflower oil rather than margarine while cooking, or have sunflower seeds rather than nut spread for a tidbit.

Utilizing Fats Astutely

You can utilize fats astutely to bring down diabetes risk and lose more weight. To begin with, pick better fat sources.

Great and bad Endlessly fat Sources
- Avocados
- Nuts, nut margarine, nut oils
- Seeds, seed margarine, seed oil
- Flaxseed and flaxseed oil
- Olive oil and vegetable oil
- Greasy fish
- French fries, broiled chicken and fish, doughnuts, and other seared food varieties
- Bundled food varieties containing, hydrogenated and to some degree hydrogenated palm oils
- Greasy red meat and skin from poultry
- Spread, fat, shortening, margarine

Then, watch your part sizes to try not to get such a large number of calories.

- 1 teaspoon of oil.
- 1 oz. of nuts, seeds, or peanuts.
- 3 oz. of greasy fish.
- 1 tablespoon of salad dressing.
- ¼ cup of avocado.

Then, at that point, eat them with nutritious food sources, like lean proteins, vegetables, natural products, or entire grains. You won't get as numerous medical advantages if you have, express, guacamole with tortilla chips, peanut butter heated into treats, soybean oil prepared into a blueberry biscuit with 40 grams of sugar, or salad dressing in a serving of mixed greens with bacon pieces, bread garnishes, and a heap of cheddar. All things being equal, you could attempt:

- Guacamole with crude vegetables.
- Prepared fish with steamed vegetables and earthy-colored rice.
- Entire wheat pasta with olive oil, tomatoes, basil, and barbecued chicken.
- Nuts and apple cuts.
- Oats with walnuts, pumpkin, and cinnamon.
- Curds with sunflower seeds.
- Prepared zucchini fries with olive oil.
- Assist with Fats

Whether you know every one of your fats as of now or you are as yet realizing what fat is, Warbler DPP is there to direct you in the correct bearing. Log your food varieties and utilize the application frequently so you can get input on the most proficient method to involve fats for your potential benefit for weight reduction and diabetes anticipation.

Chapter 6

Organizing an eating regimen for economical weight reduction

Eating fewer carbs for fat misfortune can be troublesome and nearly appear to be a ceaseless excursion, yet it unquestionably needn't bother to be if you figure out how to construct a charming and maintainable eating regimen plan.

Despite many's thought processes, weight reduction isn't generally about extreme limitations and unbending nature, yet rather tracking down ways of bettering control food admission while changing dinners to be more fitting for your objectives.

Although many individuals think radical change is required, doing so will make weight reduction considerably more troublesome and surely not pleasant.

Tracking down ways of alleviating this trouble is extremely critical for a successful eating routine.

In this article, I'll address a few key strategies I've utilized with a large number of clients throughout the years to guarantee significant weight reduction that is pleasant and economical.

Begin With An Unobtrusive Decrease Of Calories

It is no secret to prevail with a compelling eating routine, you'll have to limit calories somehow, whether by straightforwardly diminishing the calories you devour or incidentally expanding the nature of the food you eat.

This is because of the hypothesis of energy balance, expressing that to lose body weight, you want to exhaust a greater number of calories than you consume, making a negative energy balance1.

Sadly notwithstanding, many individuals move too soon and make extremely huge calorie deficiency than they need, making monstrous yearning and the impulse to stop before any significant body changes have happened.

Further, regularly when this happens, weight reduction comes to a dramatic stop, not long after the start, passing on the individual with no extra calories to confine and no extra weight reduction.

As opposed to slicing your calorie consumption down the middle, begin with a significant yet unobtrusive decrease of calories coming in at around 20% of your all-out calorie consumption. For instance, an individual consistently consuming 2000 calories ought to decrease to around 1600-1700 calories each day.

This is rather than the number of individuals that start slimming down by radically confining calories right all along.

Instead of confining every one of your calories immediately, tone it down by limiting just around 20% of calories and afterward decreasing further once weight reduction levels. Utilizing this sum will take into consideration significant weight reduction, yet give you more calories to limit when weight reduction levels.

Eat Like Your Ongoing Dietary patterns

In the wellness world, there are in a real sense many different eating fewer carbs approaches, all professing to give a similar outcome. Some emphasize limiting sugars while others center around expanding dietary fats.

In any case, it's memorable's vital that the best eating regimen is one that you'll stay steady with while having a good time.

Since an eating routine's viability relies upon your capacity to stay with it, it's constantly proposed to intently match your ongoing propensities as precisely as conceivable so that changing marginally to stick to the eating regimen will be simple and compelling.

M&S Competitor Building a Pleasant Eating routine

I've frequently been confused by how many individuals who, for instance, love to eat sugars, yet pick a low-carb ketogenic way of counting calories. Without a doubt, a low-carb-based diet will be viable however on the off chance that you're continually needing carbs, it very well may be a catastrophe waiting to happen in the long haul.

As opposed to totally evacuating your dietary patterns, attempt to track down ways of confining calorie admission, yet do as such in manners that permit you to keep eating near ordinary. Doing so will make the cycle more charming and it will likewise be almost certain that you'll adhere to it.

Keep away from Extraordinary Limitations

Many individuals' most memorable line of activity while endeavoring to get more fit is the serious limitation of specific food varieties they accept as the justification for their weight gain. Well-known substances falling into this class incorporate pop, starches, and shockingly, even good nutrition types like dairy.

Sadly, while this strategy might give starting weight reduction, at last individuals collapse and thus start to consume these items once more, generally in ludicrous sums.

The issue with this way to deal with weight reduction is that it's essentially not manageable and as a rule brings about sensations of culpability, massive enticement, and ultimately gorging.

As referenced above, energy balance is the main calculated fat misfortune. While confining utilization of food can surely assist with moving the tide in the blessing of weight reduction, that doesn't imply that you want to limit utilization completely.

For instance, decreasing non-light soft drinks is most likely smart for weight reduction and is periodically an initial step for some while shedding pounds. In any case, consider briefly that numerous soft drinks have calorie-free forms.

For this situation, essentially changing from a non-light soft drink to a calorie-free rendition will give the vital decrease of calories, yet still, take into consideration the utilization of pop.

This is without referencing that some examination shows that polishing off sugar-free refreshments may truly be more compelling for weight reduction than just drinking water alone! By exchanging the sort of pop being consumed, you'll take into consideration substances you appreciate while proceeding to wipe out the pointless calories2.

Further, while confining sugars might be a compelling way for decreasing body weight, it's anything but a necessity. Confining sugars isn't prompted except if you're wanting to utilize a ketogenic way of eating less junk food.

If you partake in specific substances, which are calorically thick, first attempt to track down ways of diminishing their caloric effect, as opposed to expecting you want to limit them. Doing so will consider more consistency to the eating regimen while making the eating regimen charming.

Make Even Cheat Feasts Valuable

While counting calories, many individuals adopt a win-big or bust strategy about the food varieties that are being eaten. Ordinarily, I've seen clients goof on their eating regimen and choose to completely leave the interaction.

Tragically for them, consuming fewer calories needn't bother with being a win big or bust approach. Rather, it's an excursion for certain great days and some terrible ones.

Rather than forcing yourself into having a not-exactly-ideal dinner and leaving the eating routine, I propose organizing your feasts as per significance, guaranteeing that even "cheat dinners' ' are gainful.

Allow me to paint a model for you.

Suppose you are keen on having some pizza for supper. Typically, individuals would simply consume five or six pieces and call it dinner. Be that as it may, assuming you want to further develop body arrangement, this is positively not an ideal dinner.

As opposed to simply eating the pizza, I propose having a little, nice dinner only before devouring the pizza, which contains protein and some type of fiber, for example, from a serving of mixed greens.

M&S Competitor Making a Cheat Dinner Useful

By devouring these fixings first, you're turning a horrible dinner (with regards to benefit) into one that is entirely balanced, containing protein, fiber, sugar, and fat, rather than a feast of just starch and fat (pizza).

Further, by devouring protein and fiber first, you'll probably eat less pizza, possibly going from five to six parts of simply a few.

Rather than projecting judgement to the breeze with regards to additional luscious food varieties, eat the fixings you want first and afterward eat the cheat dinner fixings. You'll transform an inferior dinner into a mostly fair one.

Take Standard Eating regimen Breaks

A serious mix-up many make with slimming down is continually confining calories for significant periods.

At the point when you initially start eating less junk food and limiting calories, you're consuming a greater number of calories than you eat, since your metabolic rate is still genuinely high. Sadly be that as it may, as an endurance system, your metabolic rate, at last, adjusts, stopping weight reduction.

From here, more limitation is required and in the long run, this can make unfortunate behaviour patterns seemingly forever.

As opposed to confining calories constantly, I recommend enjoying standard reprieves, utilizing what is known as refeeds to give a break to both your digestion as well as your brain research, since consuming fewer calories can frequently be unpleasant.

By enjoying customary reprieves from consuming fewer calories where you increment calories to a typical level, you offer your digestion a reprieve, guaranteeing that it doesn't adjust to the new, lower calorie consumption. Also, consuming bigger measures of calories infrequently will give a genuinely necessary break, intellectually.

M&S Competitor Setting up Certain Eggs

This isn't simply assessment either, late examination proposes that normal breaks from calorie limitation might be more gainful than continually restricting.

While executing this system, I propose enjoying some time off under two conditions. To start with, assuming that you find that weight reduction has leveled for several days, it very well may be an ideal opportunity to enjoy some time off from confining calories.

Second, having some time off in the scope of 3 a month and a half in the wake of the beginning is as yet suggested.

On the off chance that weight reduction is as yet happening, enjoying some time off may not be essential, yet it's consistently reasonable to attempt to be on the ball. Assuming that you observe that weight reduction is beginning to slow, it might be really smart to think about enjoying some time off.

By enjoying normal reprieves from calorie limitation, you'll keep away from metabolic variation while offering yourself a truly necessary reprieve from the grumbles of slimming down.

Step-by-step instructions to Fabricate A More Charming and Maintainable Eating regimen

Counting calories can some of the time feel troublesome, prohibitive, and in all honesty, a weight. Nonetheless, it needn't bother to be like that. A considerable lot of the normal entanglements individuals make while slimming down can be tried not to by track down approaches to marginally change your ongoing way of life propensities, as opposed to drastically changing them under the misrepresentation that doing so will prompt weight reduction.

By utilizing these methods, you ought to be on the way to a more charming and maintainable eating fewer carbs approach that works, and will do as such quickly.

Chapter 7

The stoutness fix diet

It's a well-known fact that how many calories individuals eat and drink straightforwardly affects their weight: Polish off the very number of calories that the body consumes over the long run, and weight stays stable. Takes more than the body takes, weight goes high. Less, weight goes down. In any case, what might be said about the kind of calories: Does it matter whether they come from explicit supplements, fat, protein, or starch? Explicit food sources entire grains or potato chips? Explicit eating regimens the Mediterranean eating regimen or the "Twinkie" diet? Also, what might be said about when or where individuals consume their calories: Does having breakfast make it simpler to control weight? Does eating at drive-through eateries make it harder?

There's more than adequate examination of food varieties and diet designs that safeguard against coronary illness, stroke, diabetes, and other persistent circumstances. Fortunately, a significant number of the food sources that assist with forestalling infection likewise appear to assist with weight control-food varieties like entire grains, vegetables, natural products, and nuts. Furthermore, a large number of the food sources that increase sickness risk-boss among them, refined grains and sweet beverages, are likewise figured to gain weight. Conventional insight expresses that since a calorie is a calorie, no matter what its source, the best guidance for weight control is just to eat less and practice more. However, rising research recommends that a few food sources and eating examples might make it simpler to hold calories under control, while others might make individuals bound to gorge.

This article momentarily audits the examination on dietary admission and weight control, featuring diet methodologies that likewise assist with forestalling persistent sickness.

Macronutrients and Weight: Do Carbohydrates, Protein, or Fat have much need?

At the point when individuals eat controlled and consume fewer calories in research center examinations, the level of calories from fat, protein, and starch doesn't appear to be an issue for weight reduction. In examinations where individuals can openly pick what they eat, there might be a few advantages to a higher protein, lower starch approach. For constant illness avoidance, however, the quality and food wellsprings of these supplements matter more than their overall amount in the eating regimen. What's more, the most recent examination recommends that a similar eating routine quality message applies to weight control.

Dietary Fat and Weight

Low-fat eating regimens have for some time been promoted as the way to a sound weight and great well-being. However, the proof simply isn't there: Throughout recent years in the U.S., the level of calories from fat in individuals' eating regimens has gone down, yet heftiness rates have soared. Painstakingly led clinical preliminaries have found that following a low-fat eating regimen doesn't make it any more straightforward to get thinner than following a moderate-or high-fat eating routine. Concentrate on volunteers who follow moderate-or high-fat eating regimens losing the same amount of weight, and in certain examinations somewhat more, as the people who follow low-fat eating regimens. And with regards to illness counteraction, low-fat eating regimens don't seem to offer any extraordinary advantages.

A contributor to the issue with low-fat eating regimens is that they are many times high in starch, particularly from quickly processed sources, like white bread and white rice. Furthermore, eating less high in such food varieties increases the gamble of weight gain, diabetes, and coronary illness. (See Carbs and Weight, underneath.)

For good well-being, the kind of husky individuals eat is undeniably more vital that the sum and there's some proof that the equivalent might be valid for weight control. In the Medical attendants' Wellbeing Study, for instance, which followed 42,000 middle-aged and more established people for a very long time, expanded utilization of undesirable fats-trans fats, particularly, yet in addition immersed fats-was connected to weight gain, yet expanded utilization of sound fats-monounsaturated and polyunsaturated fat-was not.

Protein and Weight

Higher protein eats fewer carbs appear to enjoy a few benefits for weight reduction, however more so in momentary preliminaries; in longer-term studies, high-protein counts calories appear to perform similarly well as different kinds of diets. High-protein slims down will generally be low in sugar and high in fat, so separating the advantages of eating loads of protein from those of eating more fat or less carbohydrate is troublesome. In any case, there are a couple of justifications for why eating a higher level of calories from protein might assist with weight control:

- **More satiety**: Individuals will quite often feel more full, on fewer calories, in the wake of eating protein than they do after eating sugar or fat.

- **More prominent thermic impact:** It takes more energy to use and store protein than other macronutrients, and this might assist with increasing the energy they consume every day.

- **Further developed body structure:** Protein appears to assist with people clinging to slender muscle during weight reduction, and this, as well, can assist with supporting the energy-consumed side of the energy balance condition.

Higher protein and lower carbs eating fewer carbs further develop blood lipid profiles and other metabolic markers, so they might assist with forestalling coronary illness and diabetes. Yet some high-protein food sources are more grounded than others: High admissions of red meat and handled meat is related to an expanded gamble of coronary illness, diabetes, and colon malignant growth.

Supplanting red and handled meat with nuts, beans, fish, or poultry appears to bring down the gamble of coronary illness and diabetes. And this diet system might assist with weight control, as well, as per a new report from the Harvard School of General Wellbeing. Scientists followed the eating regimen and way of life propensities for 120,000 people for as long as 20 years, seeing how little changes added to weight gain over the long run. Individuals who ate more red and handled meat throughout the review put on more weight-about a pound extra like clockwork. Individuals who ate more nuts throughout the review put on less weight-about a half pound less like clockwork.

Starches and Weight

Lower starch, higher protein diets might have some weight reduction benefits temporarily.

Yet with regards to forestalling weight gain and ongoing illness, starch quality is significantly more significant than sugar amount.

Processed, refined grains and food sources made with them-white rice, white bread, white pasta, handled breakfast cereals, and such are wealthy in quickly processed starch. Potatoes and sweet beverages are as well. The logical term for this is that they have a high glycemic file and glycemic load. Such food sources cause quick and angry expansions in glucose and insulin that, temporarily, can make hunger spike and can prompt gorging and over the long haul, increase the gamble of weight gain, diabetes, and coronary illness.

For instance, in the eating routine and way of life change study, individuals who expanded their utilization of French fries, potatoes and potato chips, sweet beverages, and refined grains put on more weight over the long run an extra 3.4, 1.3, 1.0, and 0.6 pounds like clockwork, separately. Individuals who diminished their admission of these food varieties put on less weight.

Explicit Food sources that Make It Simpler or Harder to Control Weight

There's developing proof that particular food decisions might assist with weight control. Fortunately a considerable lot of the food sources that are valuable for weight control likewise assist with forestalling coronary illness, diabetes, and other persistent infections. On the other hand, food varieties and beverages that add to weight gain boss among them, refined grains and sweet beverages likewise add to persistent sickness.

Entire grains-entire wheat, earthy colored rice, grain, and such, particularly in their less-handled structures are processed more leisurely than refined grains. So they gentler affect glucose and insulin, which might assist with keeping hunger under control. The equivalent is valid for most vegetables and natural products. These "slow carb" food sources have plentiful advantages for sickness avoidance, and there's likewise proof that they can assist with forestalling weight gain.

The weight control proof is more grounded for entire grains than it is for products of the soil.

The latest help comes from the Harvard School of General Wellbeing diet and way of life change review: Individuals who expanded their admission of entire grains, entirely natural products (not natural product juice), and vegetables throughout the 20-year concentrate on put on less weight-0.4, 0.5, and 0.2 pounds less at regular intervals, separately.

The calories from entire grains, entire organic products, and vegetables don't vanish. Reasonable happening is that when individuals increment their admission of these food sources, they cut back on calories from different food sources. Fiber might be answerable for these food sources' weight control benefits, since fiber eases back assimilation, assisting with checking hunger. Products of the soil are additionally high in water, which might assist with people feeling more full on fewer calories.

Nuts pack a lot of calories into a little bundle and are high in fat, so they were once viewed as no for weight watchers. It just so happens, investigations discover that eating nuts doesn't prompt weight gain and may rather assist with weight control, maybe because nuts are wealthy in protein and fiber, the two of which might assist with people feeling more full and less ravenous.

Individuals who routinely eat nuts are less inclined to have respiratory failures or pass on from coronary illness than the people who seldom eat them, which is one more motivation to remember nuts for a solid eating routine.

The U.S. dairy industry has forcefully advanced the weight reduction advantages of milk and other dairy items, dependent generally upon discoveries from transient investigations it has financed. Yet a new survey of almost 50 randomized preliminaries finds little proof that high dairy or calcium admissions assist with weight reduction. Comparably, most long-haul follow-up examinations have not found that dairy or calcium safeguards against weight gain, and one concentrate in teenagers viewed high milk admissions as related to expanded weight file.

One special case is the new dietary and way of life change review from the Harvard School of General Wellbeing, which found that individuals who expanded their yoghurt intake put on less weight; expansions in milk and cheddar consumption, nonetheless, didn't seem to advance weight reduction or gain.

It's conceivable that the advantageous microscopic organisms in yoghurt might impact weight control, yet more examination is required.

Sugar-Improved Refreshments and Weight

There's persuading proof that sweet beverages increase the gamble of weight gain, stoutness, and diabetes: A deliberate survey and meta-examination of 88 investigations found a "clear relationship of soda pop admission with expanded caloric admission and body weight." In kids and youths, a later meta examination gauges that for 12 extra ounces serving of sweet refreshment consumed every day, weight record increments by 0.08 units. Another meta-examination finds that grown-ups who routinely drink sugared refreshments have a 26 percent higher gamble of creating type 2 diabetes than individuals who seldom drink sugared refreshments. Arising proof likewise recommends that high sweet drink admission builds the gamble of coronary illness.

Like refined grains and potatoes, sweet drinks are high in quickly processed starch. (See Starches and Weight, above.) Exploration recommends that when that sugar is conveyed in a fluid structure, as opposed to a strong structure, it isn't as satisfying, and individuals don't eat less to make up for the additional calories.

These discoveries on sweet beverages are disturbing, considering that youngsters and grown-ups are drinking ever-bigger amounts of them: In the U.S., sugared refreshments made up around 4% of day-to-day calorie admission during the 1970s, however by 2001, addressed around 9% of calories. The latest information finds that on some random day, a big part of Americans polish off some sort of sugared refreshment, 25% polish off no less than 200 calories from sugary beverages, and 5 percent consume no less than 567 calories, which might be compared to four jars of sweet pop.

Fortunately concentrates on kids and grown-ups have additionally demonstrated the way that scaling back sweet beverages can prompt weight reduction. Sweet beverages have turned into a significant objective for corpulence avoidance endeavors, inciting conversations of strategy drives like burdening pop.

Organic product Squeeze and Weight

It's essential to take note that organic product juices are not a preferred choice for weight command over sugar-improved drinks. Ounce for ounce, natural product juices-even those that are 100% organic product juice, with no additional sugar-are as high in sugar and calories as sweet soft drinks. So it's nothing unexpected that a new Harvard School of General Wellbeing review, which followed the eating routine and way of life propensities for 120,000 people for as long as 20 years, found that individuals who expanded their admission of organic product juice put on more weight after some time than individuals who didn't. Paediatricians and general well-being advocates suggest that youngsters and grown-ups limit natural product juice to simply a little glass a day, on the off chance that they drink it by any means.

Although most cocktails have a greater number of calories per ounce than sugar-improved refreshments, there's no obvious proof that moderate drinking adds to weight gain. While the new eating regimen and way of life change investigation discovered that individuals who expanded their liquor consumption put on more weight after some time, the discoveries shifted by kind of liquor.

In many past planned examinations, there was no distinction in weight gain after some time between light-to-direct consumers and nondrinkers, or the light-to-direct consumers put on less weight than non-drinkers.

Diet Examples, Part Size, and Weight

Individuals don't eat supplements or food sources in separation. They eat dinners that fall into a general eating example, and specialists have started investigating whether specific eating routines or feast designs assist with weight control or add to weight gain. Segment sizes have additionally expanded emphatically throughout recent many years, as has utilization of inexpensive food-U.S.

kids, for instance, devour a more prominent level of calories from inexpensive food than they do from school food and these patterns are likewise remembered to be supporters of the heftiness pandemic.

Dietary Examples and Weight

Purported "reasonable" dietary examples abstain from food that highlight entire grains, vegetables, and natural products appear to safeguard against weight gain, though "Western-style" dietary examples with more red meat or handled meat, sugared drinks, desserts, refined carbs, or potatoes-have been connected to stoutness. The Western-style dietary example is likewise connected to the expanded hazard of coronary illness, diabetes, and other persistent circumstances.

Following a Mediterranean-style diet, proven and factual to safeguard against constant sickness, has all the earmarks of being promising for weight control, as well. The customary Mediterranean-style diet is higher in fat (around 40% of calories) than the normal American eating routine (34% of calories), however, a large portion of the fat comes from olive oil and other plant sources. The eating routine is likewise wealthy in natural products, vegetables, nuts, beans, and fish. A 2008 precise survey viewed that as in the vast majority of studies, individuals who followed a Mediterranean-style diet had lower paces of corpulence or more weight reduction. There is no single "Mediterranean" diet, in any case, and concentrates frequently utilize various definitions, so more exploration is required.

Breakfast, Dinner Recurrence, Nibbling, and Weight

There is some proof that skipping breakfast expands the gamble of weight gain and corpulence, however, the proof is more grounded in youngsters, particularly adolescents than it is in grown-ups. Dinner recurrence and eating have expanded throughout recent years in the U.S. (overall, youngsters get 27% of their everyday calories from snacks, essentially from treats and sweet beverages, and progressively from pungent tidbits and candy. Be that as it may, there have been clashing discoveries on the connection between feast recurrence, nibbling, and weight control, and more exploration is required.

Segment Sizes and Weight

Since the 1970s, segment sizes have expanded both for food eaten at home and for food consumed from home, in grown-ups and youngsters. Momentary investigations exhibit that when individuals are served bigger segments, they eat more. One review, for instance, gave moviegoers compartments of old popcorn in one or the other enormous or medium-sized cans; individuals announced that they could have done without the flavor of the popcorn-and all things considered, the people who got huge holders ate around 30% more popcorn than the individuals who got medium-sized compartments.

Another review showed that individuals given bigger refreshments would in general drink fundamentally more, however, didn't diminish their ensuing food utilization. An extra review furnished proof that when given bigger piece sizes, individuals would in general eat more, with no reduction in later food consumption.

There is a natural enticement for the possibility that part measures increment corpulence, however long-haul imminent examinations would assist with reinforcing this speculation.

Cheap Food and Weight

Cheap food is known for its enormous segments, low costs, high acceptability, and high sugar content, and there's proof from concentrates on adolescents and grown-ups that continuous inexpensive food utilization adds to gorging and weight gain. The CARDIA study, for instance, followed 3,000 youthful grown-ups for a long time. Individuals who had higher inexpensive food consumption levels toward the beginning of the review gauged a normal of around 13 pounds more than individuals who had the most reduced cheap food-admission levels.

They likewise had bigger midsection boundaries and more prominent expansions in triglycerides, and twofold the chances of creating metabolic disorder. More examination is expected to prod separated the impact of eating cheap food itself from the impact on the local individuals' lives, or other individual characteristics that might make individuals bound to eat inexpensive food.

The Reality: Sound Eating regimen Can Forestall Weight Gain and Constant Sickness
Weight gain in adulthood is in many cases progressive, about a pound a year excessively

delayed of an addition for the vast majority to see, however, one that can add up, over the long run, to a profound individual and general medical condition. There's rising proof that similar stimulating food decisions and diet designs that assist with forestalling coronary illness, diabetes, and other constant circumstances may likewise assist with forestalling weight gain:

Pick negligibly handled, entire food sources entire grains, vegetables, natural products, nuts, stimulating wellsprings of protein (fish, poultry, beans), and plant oils.

Limit sugared drinks, refined grains, potatoes, red and handled meats, and other profoundly handled food sources, like inexpensive food.

However the commitment of anyone eating regimen change to weight control might be little, together, the progressions could amount to a significant impact, after some time and across the entire society. Since individuals' food decisions are molded by their environmental elements, states must advance arrangements and natural changes that make good food sources more open and reduce the accessibility and showcasing of unhealthful food varieties.

Conclusion

Treating Obesity

The most effective way to treat weight is to eat a solid, diminished-calorie diet and work out routinely. To do this you ought to:

eat a decent, calorie-controlled diet as suggested by your GP or weight reduction the board well-being proficient (like a dietitian)

join a nearby weight reduction bunch

take up exercises, for example, quick strolling, running, swimming, or tennis for 150 to 300 minutes (over two to five hours) seven days

eat gradually and stay away from circumstances where you realize you could be enticed to gorge

You may likewise profit from getting mental help from a prepared medical service proficient to assist with having an impact on how you contemplate food and eating.

If the way of life changes alone don't assist you with getting more fit, a prescription called orlistat might be suggested. Whenever taken accurately, this medicine works by decreasing how much fat you assimilate during processing. Your GP will know whether orlistat is appropriate for you.

In uncommon cases, weight reduction medical procedures might be suggested.